ICD-O

International Classification of Diseases for Oncology

FIRST EDITION
1976

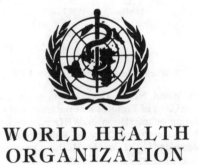

WORLD HEALTH ORGANIZATION
Geneva, Switzerland

ISBN   92 4 154056 7

PRINTED IN SWITZERLAND

CONTENTS

PREFACE

The *International Classification of Diseases for Oncology* (ICD-O) represents an extension of Chapter II (Neoplasms) of the Ninth Revision of the *International Classification of Diseases* (ICD-9). ICD-O permits the coding of all neoplasms by topography, histology (morphology) and behavior; i.e., malignant, benign, in-situ, of uncertain behavior, or metastatic. A separate code for histologic grading and differentiation has also been included. Thus ICD-O is a coded nomenclature which can be used for both topographic sites and histologic types of neoplasms by those who wish to code greater detail about a neoplasm than is provided for in the neoplasms chapter of ICD-9. It does not provide codes for other types of information such as staging, extent of disease, laterality, method of diagnosis and treatment.

For many years the *International Classification of Diseases* (ICD) has been used throughout the world by the Member States of the World Health Organization to code and tabulate mortality and morbidity statistics. More recently, ICD has also been used to code hospital and other medical records for purposes of storage and retrieval.

Since the Sixth Revision (1948), neoplasms have been classified in Chapter II of ICD, the classification being largely based on the topographic sites of tumors and on whether they are malignant or benign. Except for lymphatic and hematopoietic neoplasms, choriocarcinoma, malignant melanoma and certain benign neoplasms, there has been no coded nomenclature for histologic types.

In 1968, the International Agency for Research on Cancer (IARC) was asked by WHO to make recommendations about the content and structure of Chapter II of ICD-9 in consultation with the Cancer and ICD units of WHO and various national bodies. A large number of consultants and committees from various countries collaborated with the working parties appointed by IARC to make suggestions for Chapter II of ICD-9. These working parties, recognizing a worldwide need for a detailed and uniform histopathology code for neoplasms, proposed that WHO should publish a coded nomenclature for the histology of neoplasms as a supplement to Chapter II in ICD-9. After examining several coding schemes, they recommended that the proposed code should be based on the morphology section of the *Manual of Tumor Nomenclature and Coding* (MOTNAC)[1] which, in turn, was based on the Eighth Revision of ICD and the *Systematized Nomenclature of Pathology* (SNOP)[2]. MOTNAC has received a wide measure of international acceptance and has been translated into French, Italian, Japanese, Portuguese and Spanish.

The working parties further recommended that for the use of specialists in oncology who require greater detail of histologic classification, a special adaptation, to be designated ICD-O, be created as the successor to MOTNAC. This recommendation was endorsed by a Study Group on Classification of Diseases convened by WHO in 1971.

In developing the morphology section of ICD-O, a particular effort was made to stress the histologic terms for neoplasms listed in the *International Histological Classification of Tumours* series (*"Blue Books"*) published by WHO. These classifications are the result of a major international effort to develop uniform criteria for the histologic definition, nomenclature and classification of neoplasms. The importance of this effort is emphasized in the general preface to the series which includes the statement: "An internationally agreed classification of tumours, acceptable alike to physicians, surgeons, radiologists, pathologists and statisticians, would enable cancer workers in all parts of the world to compare their findings and would facilitate collaboration among them".

In 1975 and 1976, a series of field trials were conducted in many countries to test the new ICD-O. Approximately 35,000 records pertaining to the diagnosis of neoplasms were coded. Included were

---

[1]Manual of Tumor Nomenclature and Coding, New York, N.Y., American Cancer Society, Inc. (1968).

[2]Systematized Nomenclature of Pathology, Chicago, Ill., College of American Pathologists (1965).

records from population-based cancer registries and hospital registries, from pathology and clinical departments and from death certificates. A particular effort was made to include records of neoplasms from various specialties such as dermatology, pediatrics, oral pathology and gynecology. The experience from coding this large number of records and the results of data retrieval and analysis of the coded records were used in the final editing of ICD-O. The assistance of pathologists, epidemiologists, cancer registrars, medical record librarians, and statisticians who participated in these field trials is gratefully acknowledged.

While taking into account user needs and current concepts of morphology and histogenesis, the committees have constantly kept in mind the need to preserve as much continuity as possible with previous ICD revisions and MOTNAC.

It is hoped that ICD-O will serve to promote international cooperation in the field of cancer in accordance with resolution WHA 28.85[3] of the Twenty-eighth World Health Assembly in 1975, which requested the Director-General "to consider . . . steps to fulfil the need to accelerate . . . international coordination of cancer research and the elaboration of information systems . . . to support the comprehensive cancer research programme, taking into account the proposals of national and international organizations interested in participation in this programme."

[3] Off. Rec., Wld Hlth Org., 1975, 226, 50.

WORKING PARTIES AND COMMITTEES FOR DEVELOPMENT OF ICD-O

A number of working parties and committees constituted by WHO and IARC contributed to the preparation of ICD-O. The following have participated in the work of these committees either as members or as expert consultants:

Professor G. Avtandilov, Moscow, USSR
Dr J.W. Berg, Iowa City, Iowa, USA
Mrs R. Carleschi, London, United Kingdom
Mr H.G. Corbett, WHO
Dr U. de Jong, IARC
Dr J. Delafresnaye, UICC
Mrs A. Dolman, Rockville, Md., USA
Dr R. Gerard-Marchant, Paris, France
Dr P. Graepel, Bethesda, Md., USA
Dr D.E. Henson, Bethesda, Md., USA
Dr K. Kupka, WHO
Mr A. L'Hours, WHO
Mr W.I. Lourie, Jr., Bethesda, Md., USA
Miss R.M. Loy, London, United Kingdom
Dr C.S. Muir, IARC
Dr N.P. Napalkov, Leningrad, USSR

Mrs J. Nectoux, IARC
Dr G.T. O'Conor, Bethesda, Md., USA
Mr H.G. Page, Ottawa, Canada
Dr E. Pedersen, Oslo, Norway
Mrs C. Percy, Bethesda, Md., USA
Dr F. Rilke, Milan, Italy
Dr A.H.T. Robb-Smith, Oxford, United Kingdom
Dr A.A. Romensky, Moscow, USSR
Dr A. Rothschild, Paris, France
Dr E. Saxén, Helsinki, Finland
Dr L. Sobin, WHO
Dr L.B. Thomas, Bethesda, Md., USA
Dr H. Tulinius, IARC
Dr G. Wagner, Heidelberg, Federal Republic of Germany
Dr A. Winkler, WHO

The members of these working parties and committees could not have worked effectively without the support and interest of many individual expert consultants from specialty groups, cancer registries and national offices of vital statistics who commented on various proposals and drafts and whose experience contributed to the development of ICD-O. Special acknowledgement should be made of the contributions of Dr. Peter H. Graepel, Dr. Donald E. Henson, Mrs. Constance L. Percy and Dr. Louis B. Thomas, who served as the editorial subcommittee for the final preparation of the present edition as well as the field trial version. Computer programs and assistance were generously provided by the staff of the Biometry Branch, National Cancer Institute, and the Division of Computer Research and Technology, National Institutes of Health, Bethesda, Md., USA.

The project was supported in part by a contract (NO1-CO-55218) from the National Cancer Institute, National Institutes of Health, Bethesda, Md., USA.

INTRODUCTION

STRUCTURE

The *International Classification of Diseases for Oncology* (ICD-O) consists of three main sections:

(1) Topography - Numerical List

The topography section has been adapted from the malignant neoplasms section of Chapter II of ICD-9. The topography terms have 4-digit code numbers which run from 140.0 to 199.9. A decimal point (.) indicates subdivisions of the 3-digit rubrics.

(2) Morphology - Numerical List

The morphology section is a revised and expanded version of the morphology section of the *Manual of Tumor Nomenclature and Coding*, 1968 Edition (MOTNAC). The morphology terms have 5-digit code numbers which run from 8000/0 to 9990/6; the first four digits indicate the specific histologic terms and the fifth digit, after the slash mark or solidus (/), is a behavior code.

(3) Alphabetic Index

The alphabetic index, which is to be used primarily for coding, includes topography (anatomical sites), morphology (histologic terms) and selected tumor-like lesions and conditions.

The numerical lists display the structure of the coded nomenclature and constitute the primary point of reference for retrieval or decoding.

There is a separate code for histologic grading and differentiation. Therefore 10 digits are necessary for the complete identification of topographic site, morphologic type, behavior, and grade or differentiation of a neoplasm.

Abbreviations

The following abbreviations are used throughout:

T - **Topography**

M - **Morphology**

NOS - Not Otherwise Specified

Format of ICD-O Terms

Each topographic and morphologic term appears only once in the numerical list. The first listed term under a particular code number (rubric) is either the preferred term or an inclusive term appropriate for retrieval and is printed in bold type.

Example:

194.0 Suprarenal gland
Adrenal gland
Adrenal, NOS
Adrenal cortex
Adrenal medulla

In this example, "Suprarenal gland" would describe all cases coded to T-194.0. The synonyms, "Adrenal gland" and "Adrenal, NOS", are indented under "Suprarenal gland". The non-indented terms," Adrenal cortex" and "Adrenal medulla", are not synonyms but are listed under the same code number because they are topographic subdivisions of the term printed first, "Suprarenal gland". In the alphabetic index all these terms are given the code number T-194.0.

Meaning of "NOS"

"NOS" is printed after topographic and morphologic terms that appear elsewhere in ICD-O with some modifying word or phrase. In the alphabetic index "NOS" is listed first followed by the alphabetic listing of modifying words. The code number for a term followed by "NOS" should be used when a topographic or morphologic term is not modified or when it has an adjective that does not appear elsewhere in ICD-O. For example, in the alphabetic index, "Adenocarcinoma, NOS" is followed by a long list of adjectives, each with their specific code numbers:

	Adenocarcinoma *(see also Carcinoma)*
M-8140/3	NOS
M-8140/6	NOS, metastatic
M-8280/3	acidophil
M-8550/3	acinar
M-8550/3	acinic cell
M-8370/3	adrenal cortical
M-8251/3	alveolar
M-8560/3	and epidermoid carcinoma, mixed
M-8560/3	and squamous cell carcinoma, mixed
M-8401/3	apocrine
M-8300/3	basophil
M-8160/3	bile duct
M-8250/3	bronchiolar
M-8250/3	bronchiolo-alveolar
M-8420/3	ceruminous
M-8270/3	chromophobe

etc.

If the diagnosis is "Adenocarcinoma", the correct code is M-8140/3 "Adenocarcinoma, NOS". If a diagnostic phrase such as "Atypical adenocarcinoma" is used, the code number is also M-8140/3 because the adjective, "Atypical", does not appear in the list of terms modifying "Adenocarcinoma". Thus, "NOS" is printed in both the numerical lists and the alphabetic index to indicate to the coder and to the decoder that other modifiers of the term are listed elsewhere. In this sense "NOS", as used in ICD-O, has a meaning equivalent to the abbreviation "NEC" (Not Elsewhere Classified) which is used in the ICD-9 index volume.

In a few instances "NOS" is also used to indicate that a particular term is used in a general sense.

For example, "NOS" is printed after "Endocrine gland"—"T-194.9 Endocrine gland, NOS"—to indicate that other specific endocrine glands such as "Pineal gland" and "Pituitary gland" are also listed with their specific code numbers.

American and English spelling

In order to avoid repetitions caused by differences in spelling, the American spelling of words, e.g., "leukemia" and "tumor" rather than "leukaemia" and "tumour", has been used. These examples do not present a serious problem in alphabetization. However, when the differences in spelling, e.g., "esophagus" and "oesophagus" result in an appreciable separation of the two forms in the alphabetic index, the reader seeking the English spelling is referred to the American by the entry, "Oesophagus (see Esophagus)".

TOPOGRAPHY

Relationship of ICD-O to ICD-9 and MOTNAC

In ICD-O, the topography code numbers or rubrics 140.0 to 199.9 are based on the malignant neoplasms section of Chapter II of ICD-9 as the topography code in MOTNAC was based on ICD-8. These topography code numbers are used to record the site of origin of all neoplasms: malignant, benign, in-situ, or uncertain whether benign or malignant. The topography code numbers in ICD-O can also be used to code the site of metastatic tumors.

ICD-9 rubrics not used in ICD-O

The rubrics (200.0 to 239.9) of other sections of Chapter II of ICD-9 are not in ICD-O because the neoplasms coded to these rubrics are completely characterized by the morphology and behavior code numbers in ICD-O combined with appropriate topography code numbers. The following sections in Chapter II of ICD-9 were thus omitted from ICD-O:

200-208	Malignant neoplasms of lymphatic and haematopoietic tissue
210-229	Benign neoplasms
230-234	Carcinoma-in-situ
235-238	Neoplasms of uncertain behaviour
239	Neoplasms of unspecified nature

The 200-208 section of ICD-9 is used for malignant neoplasms stated or presumed to be primary in lymphatic or hematopoietic tissue. These are coded in ICD-O by their specific morphology code number and the behavior code /3, combined with the appropriate topography codes 140-199. For benign neoplasms (210-229 in ICD-9) the behavior code /0 in ICD-O is used together with the appropriate topography code numbers. In-situ neoplasms (230-234 in ICD-9) are coded by the behavior code /2; and /1 is used to designate neoplasms of uncertain behavior or unspecified nature (235-239 in ICD-9). The behavior code /3 is used in ICD-O for all primary malignant neoplasms, and /6 is used to code metastatic neoplasms.

The ICD-9 rubrics 140-199 themselves include a few categories based on morphology and behavior and these categories are also omitted from ICD-O because they are identified in ICD-O by morphology and behavior codes. These ICD-9 categories which are not used in ICD-O are:

155.2	Malignant neoplasm of liver, not specified as primary or secondary
172	Malignant melanoma of skin
197	Secondary malignant neoplasm of respiratory and digestive systems
198	Secondary malignant neoplasm of other specified sites

Rubrics 196, 159.1 and 169

In ICD-9, the rubric 196 is used only for secondary and unspecified malignant neoplasms of lymph nodes, but the corresponding ICD-O code number T-196.__ is used for both primary and metastatic neoplasms of lymph nodes. Thus most of the malignant lymphomas (200-202 in ICD-9) are coded to the topography code number T-196.__ in ICD-O.

The ICD-9 rubric 159.1 for "Malignant neoplasm of spleen, NEC" does not appear in ICD-O which uses a different code number for the spleen (T-169.2). The rubric 169.__ is not used in ICD-9 but in ICD-O is used to designate several topographic sites within the hematopoietic and reticuloendothelial systems. These code numbers are used for the topography sites for most of the leukemias and related conditions which are coded to rubrics 203 to 208 in ICD-9. The listing for 169.__ in ICD-O is as follows:

169 HEMATOPOIETIC AND RETICULOENDOTHELIAL SYSTEMS

169.0 Blood
169.1 Bone marrow
169.2 Spleen
169.3 Reticuloendothelial system, NOS
169.9 Hematopoietic system, NOS

Hydatidiform mole

The final difference between ICD-O and Chapter II of ICD-9 is that "Hydatidiform mole, NOS", T-181.9 M-9100/0 in ICD-O, is not classified in Chapter II (Neoplasms) of ICD-9 but in Chapter XI "Complications of pregnancy, childbirth and the puerperium" (rubric 630).

4-Digit subdivisions of topography

The topography section of MOTNAC, which was based on the malignant neoplasms section of ICD-8, was expanded by the inclusion of additional 4-digit subdivisions. This was accomplished by dropping residual ICD-8 categories and distributing the content to unused 4-digit numbers within the same ICD-8 3-digit category. For example, in ICD-8, 157.0 was "Head of pancreas", 157.8 "Other specified parts of pancreas (body, neck and tail)" and 157.9 was "Pancreas, unspecified". In MOTNAC and in ICD-O and ICD-9, the "Body of the pancreas" and the "Tail of the pancreas" are given specific 4-digit code numbers, 157.1 and 157.2 respectively. In addition in ICD-O, the "Pancreatic ducts" are given the number 157.3, and the "Islets of Langerhans" are coded 157.4. In general, the expansions developed for MOTNAC have been incorporated into ICD-9 and then into ICD-O. Thus, there is a high order of compatibility between the topographic classification of ICD-9 and ICD-O and that of ICD-8 and MOTNAC. To achieve this degree of compatibility was considered important because hundreds of thousands of tumor diagnoses have been coded to ICD-8 and MOTNAC during the past ten years. In developing ICD-9 and ICD-O further expansions were made of some of the basic 3-digit topography rubrics by assigning new topography terms to unused 4-digit numbers. This was preferable to renumbering all the topographic sites already coded in ICD-8 and MOTNAC.

Topographic regions and ill-defined sites

The coding of diagnoses referring to regions and ill-defined sites of the body presents problems. Most of these ill-defined sites are listed under T-195.__ in ICD-O. Many of them have several component tissues and the diagnostic statement may not indicate in which tissue the tumor originated. For example, "Ankle" may refer to "Skin of ankle", to various "Soft tissues of the ankle" or even to the "Bones of the ankle". "Ankle, NOS" is given the topography code number T-195.5. To facilitate coding of tumors of the "Ankle", specific tissues of the ankle are listed below the term, "Ankle", in the alphabetic index. In addition, examples of common benign or malignant neoplasms have been listed in parentheses and assigned to the specific tissue of the "Ankle" from which these tumor types usually arise. Thus "Ankle" in the alphabetic index is listed as follows:

	Ankle
T-195.5	NOS
T-173.7	NOS (carcinoma, melanoma, nevus)
T-171.3	NOS (sarcoma, lipoma)
T-170.8	bone
T-171.3	connective tissue
T-171.3	fibrous tissue
T-170.8	joint
T-173.7	skin
T-171.3	soft tissue
T-171.3	subcutaneous tissue
T-171.3	tendon
T-171.3	tendon sheath

"Carcinoma", "Melanoma" and "Nevus" of the "Ankle" have been assigned to T-173.7, the code number which includes "Skin of ankle". These were inserted to assist the coder and indicate that various types of carcinomas of the "Ankle", such as squamous cell carcinoma or epidermoid carcinoma, should be coded to the "Skin of the ankle" T-173.7 rather than "Ankle, NOS" T-195.5.

Similarly, "Sarcoma" and "Lipoma" have been assigned to T-171.3, the code number for various soft tissues of the ankle. Most sarcomas such as fibrosarcoma, liposarcoma and angiosarcoma usually originate in soft tissue. However, osteosarcomas and chondrosarcomas usually arise in bone. "Bone of ankle" is given the code number T-170.8, which designates "Short bones of lower limb and associated joints" and is the correct code number if the osteosarcoma or chondrosarcoma arises in one of the bones of the foot. However, more information should be obtained before coding a diagnosis such as "Osteosarcoma of the ankle" because the osteosarcoma may in fact be arising in the lower end of the tibia or fibula and the correct code number for these bones is 170.7, "Long bones of lower limb and associated joints".

An approach similar to that outlined for "Ankle" was followed in the alphabetic index for other ill-defined sites and regions of the body which are listed under topography code numbers 195.0 to 195.8. A few other ill-defined sites are listed under skin; e.g., "Chin, NOS" T-173.3, because most neoplasms which might be recorded as "Chin, NOS" are in fact neoplasms arising in the "Skin of the chin".

Divisions of the esophagus

Two incompatible systems are widely used to subdivide the esophagus. Both are included in ICD-O and ICD-9, the wording in ICD-O being as follows:

150 ESOPHAGUS

150.0 Cervical esophagus

150.1 Thoracic esophagus

150.2 Abdominal esophagus

150.3 Upper third of esophagus
      Proximal third of esophagus

150.4 Middle third of esophagus

150.5 Lower third of esophagus
      Distal third of esophagus

150.8 *(See note page 1)*

150.9 Esophagus, NOS

Branchial cleft and Meckel's diverticulum as sites of neoplasms

These two terms were added to the topography section in ICD-O to provide for the coding of certain neoplasms which might originate in these congenital anomalies. The phrase "site of neoplasm" was added in parentheses after each term to indicate that they were to be used only for the site of origin of a neoplasm. Both "Meckel's diverticulum" and "Branchial cleft" are congenital abnormalities and as such are coded to rubrics 751.0 and 744.4 respectively in ICD-9. Thus the ICD-O topography numbers should not be used for these congenital anomalies unless a neoplasm arises in them.

Adjectival forms

The topographic site of a neoplasm may be denoted by use of the noun or by the related adjective, e.g., "glioma of pons" or "pontine glioma". In general, noun forms appear in the numerical list and alphabetic index of ICD-O. For example, "pons" is listed in ICD-O but "pontine" is not listed. Only a few of the commonly encountered adjectives, e.g., "uterine" and "gastric", have been listed in ICD-O for the convenience of coders.

Prefixes

The prefixes, peri-, para-, pre-, supra-, infra-, etc., are often used with topographic sites and various organs of the body. A few topographic sites modified by such prefixes are listed in ICD-O and given specific code numbers. For example, "Periadrenal tissue", "Peripancreatic tissue" and "Retrocecal tissue", are listed and given the code number T-158.0 which is "Retroperitoneum". "Para-aortic lymph node" is listed in ICD-O and given the same code number, T-196.2, as "Aortic lymph node". It is not possible to list all topographic sites which might be modified by these prefixes in ICD-O. In practice use of such prefixes indicates that the topographic site is ill-defined. Therefore it is suggested that T-195.__ should be used for such ill-defined sites not listed in ICD-O. The same general rule should also be used for other imprecise designations such as in the "area of" or in the "region of" a topographic site.

MORPHOLOGY

In developing the morphology section every effort was made to include the terms for different types of neoplasms which have been defined and illustrated in widely accepted publications of tumor classifications and which are in general usage throughout the world. In several instances the terms for neoplasms from more than one classification scheme have been included. This is illustrated by the listing of terms for the malignant lymphomas (M-959 to M-975) and for the germ cell tumors of the testis (M-906 to M-909). ICD-O is, in fact, a coded nomenclature and not a classification scheme for tumors. The listing of terms from different classifications does not represent endorsement of any particular classification scheme. In the numerical list of morphology, the first term listed under a particular code number is usually the preferred term in the *International Histological Classification of Tumours*.

Expansion of MOTNAC morphology code numbers

As noted in the Preface, the morphology section of MOTNAC was revised and expanded by the addition of many terms for more detailed histologic types and subtypes of neoplasms to create the morphology section of ICD-O. This expansion necessitated the use of an additional digit in the morphology code numbers in ICD-O. To illustrate this expansion, the MOTNAC and ICD-O entries for various types of "Squamous cell carcinoma" are compared:

MOTNAC	ICD-O
8073 Squamous cell carcinoma, NOS Epidermoid carcinoma, NOS Cancroid Acanthoma, malignant Prickle cell carcinoma Spinous cell carcinoma Squamous carcinoma	**8070/3 Squamous cell carcinoma, NOS** Epidermoid carcinoma, NOS Spinous cell carcinoma Squamous carcinoma Squamous cell epithelioma
	8071/3 Squamous cell carcinoma, keratinizing type, NOS Squamous cell carcinoma, large cell, keratinizing type Epidermoid carcinoma, keratinizing type
	8072/3 Squamous cell carcinoma, large cell, non-keratinizing type Squamous cell carcinoma, non-keratinizing type, NOS Epidermoid carcinoma, large cell, non-keratinizing type
	8073/3 Squamous cell carcinoma, small cell, non-keratinizing type Epidermoid carcinoma, small cell, non-keratinizing type
	8074/3 Squamous cell carcinoma, spindle cell type Epidermoid carcinoma, spindle cell type
	8075/3 Adenoid squamous cell carcinoma Pseudoglandular squamous cell carcinoma

In MOTNAC, "Squamous cell carcinoma, NOS" has the 4-digit code number 8073; 807 signifies the histologic type and the 4th digit "3" indicates behavior. In ICD-O, the same term has the 5-digit number 8070/3; 8070 signifies the histologic type and the 5th digit "/3" indicates behavior. The expansion to a 5-digit code for "Squamous cell carcinoma, NOS" in ICD-O was accomplished by inserting the digit "0" before the slash mark or solidus. If this added digit "0" were eliminated or disregarded, the numerical code numbers for "Squamous cell carcinoma, NOS" in MOTNAC and in ICD-O would be the same; i.e., 8073 in MOTNAC and 807_/3 in ICD-O. Additional digits, 1, 2, 3, etc., were inserted before the slash mark in the ICD-O code numbers to designate subtypes of "Squamous cell carcinoma" which were added in ICD-O but which were not listed in MOTNAC. Thus, 8071/3 is the code number assigned to "Squamous cell carcinoma, keratinizing type, NOS" and 8072/3 is the code number of "Squamous cell carcinoma, large cell, non-keratinizing type", etc. It is apparent from this scheme, that all the types or subtypes of "Squamous cell carcinoma" coded in ICD-O could contract into the 4-digit code number of MOTNAC by eliminating the new digit which has been inserted before the slash mark in the 5-digit code numbers of ICD-O. Thus, most of the additional coded terms in ICD-O represent subdivisions of histologic terms in MOTNAC and their 5-digit code numbers in ICD-O can be readily converted to the original 4-digit code numbers for these terms in MOTNAC.

In the example of "Squamous cell carcinoma, NOS" given above there are 6 synonyms under 8073 in MOTNAC and only 4 synonyms under 8070/3 "Squamous cell carcinoma, NOS" in ICD-O. Three of the MOTNAC synonyms, "Cancroid", "Acanthoma, malignant" and "Prickle cell carcinoma", were considered to be obsolete or not desirable and therefore were not included in ICD-O. Elimination of obsolete or undesirable terms does not in any way produce incompatibility between MOTNAC code numbers and ICD-O code numbers.

A few histologic terms in ICD-O have been assigned code numbers different from those in MOTNAC so that some incompatibility between the code numbers of MOTNAC and the code numbers of ICD-O has resulted but every effort was made to keep these changes to a minimum. At a later date it is planned that conversion tables will be prepared for converting data from ICD-O code numbers to MOTNAC code numbers and to ICD-9 rubrics.

Behavior code in morphology

In a morphology code number the 5th digit, which appears after the slash mark (solidus), is the behavior code. The 5th digit behavior code numbers used in ICD-O are listed below:

5th DIGIT BEHAVIOR CODE FOR NEOPLASMS

/0 .... Benign

/1 .... Uncertain whether benign or malignant
Borderline malignancy

/2 .... Carcinoma-in-situ
Intraepithelial
Non-infiltrating
Non-invasive

/3 .... Malignant, primary site

/6 .... Malignant, metastatic site
Secondary site

/9 .... Malignant, uncertain whether primary or metastatic site

For example, in the code 8070/3, which is the morphology code for "Squamous cell carcinoma, NOS", the "/3" signifies a primary, malignant neoplasm. The diagnostic phrase "Metastatic squamous cell carcinoma in the liver" would have the code numbers T-155.0 M-8070/6; the "/6" indicating the fact of metastasis. Thus, a "metastasis", or as sometimes designated a "secondary", of any of the malignant tumors listed in ICD-O can be properly coded by substituting "/6" for the "/3" in the morphology code numbers. Below is a list of several examples of the use of "/6" in morphology code numbers. Among these examples, only the first one, "Metastatic carcinoma, NOS" (8010/6), is listed in ICD-O, but all of them represent appropriate use of the "/6" to signify that a particular type of neoplasm is "metastatic" or "secondary" in a particular topographic site.

8010/3 Carcinoma, NOS
8010/6 Metastatic (or secondary) carcinoma

8720/3 Malignant melanoma, NOS
8720/6 Metastatic (or secondary) malignant
        melanoma

9180/3 Osteosarcoma, NOS
9180/6 Metastatic (or secondary) osteosarcoma

Table 1. Morphology and Behavior Code Matrix

Examples of 4-digit morphology code numbers	5th Digit behavior code numbers		
	/0 Benign	/1 Uncertain whether benign or malignant Borderline malignancy	/2 Carcinoma-in-situ Intraepithelial Non-infiltrating Non-invasive
(a) 8140	8140/0 Adenoma, NOS	8140/1 Bronchial adenoma (T-162._)	8140/2 Adenocarcinoma-in-situ
(b) 9000	9000/0 Brenner tumor, NOS	9000/1 Brenner tumor, borderline malignancy	9000/2
(c) 9370	9370/0	9370/1	9370/2

Morphology code matrix (Table 1)

The morphology code numbers for terms in ICD-O can be more completely understood by listing examples in a matrix form as shown in Table 1. In the first example (a) are 5 terms with their morphology code numbers as printed in ICD-O. "Adenoma, NOS" is a benign tumor and has the behavior code "/0". "Adenocarcinoma, NOS" is the malignant equivalent of "Adenoma, NOS" and has the behavior code "/3." "Adenocarcinoma-in-situ" has the appropriate behavior code "/2". "Bronchial adenoma" was originally described as a benign tumor but later was discovered to be malignant or potentially malignant. "Bronchial adenoma, NOS" therefore, has been assigned the behavior code "/1" to indicate that it is uncertain whether a particular bronchial adenoma will behave in a benign or malignant manner. "Metastatic adenocarcinoma, NOS" has the code number 8140/6. Each of these 5 terms has the same 4-digit morphology code number, 8140. The code number 8140/9 is also listed in the matrix even though it is not printed in the numerical list or alphabetic index of ICD-O. 8140/9 could be used for the diagnosis, "Adenocarcinoma, uncertain whether primary or metastatic site", when this diagnosis occurs in clinical or pathology records.

In the second example in the matrix, (b), there are 3 terms listed under the 4-digit morphology code number, 9000. "Brenner tumor, NOS" is usually benign, so it was assigned the code number, 9000/0. If, however, the diagnosis "Malignant Brenner tumor" is encountered, its correct code number is 9000/3 and, similarly a diagnosis of "Brenner tumor, borderline malignancy" would be correctly coded 9000/1. The code numbers 9000/2, 9000/6 and 9000/9 have not been used in ICD-O. They are available for appropriate diagnoses, e.g., 9000/6 would be used for "Metastatic Brenner tumor".

In the third example, (c), only one term, "Chordoma", is listed. "Chordoma" is usually considered to be a malignant neoplasm and is therefore assigned the morphology code number 9370/3. Other numbers in the 9370 matrix code are available and could be used for appropriate diagnoses; e.g., 9370/0 for "Benign chordoma" and 9370/6 for "Metastatic chordoma", even though these terms are not actually listed in ICD-O.

5th Digit behavior code numbers

/3 Malignant, primary site	/6 Malignant, metastatic site Secondary site	/9 Malignant, uncertain whether primary or metastatic site
8140/3 Adenocarcinoma, NOS	8140/6 Adenocarcinoma, metastatic	8140/9
9000/3 Malignant Brenner tumor	9000/6	9000/9
9370/3 Chordoma	9370/6	9370/9

Usually a term carries a clear implication as to its behavior, whether malignant or benign, and this is reflected in the behavior code number assigned to it in ICD-O. However, in the examples given in the matrix above not all possible combinations of terms have been listed for each 4-digit code number. In fact, some of the possible combinations of terms probably do not exist or have not been recognized and defined. Only a few histologic types of in-situ neoplasms are actually listed in ICD-O. The behavior code number "/2" could be attached to any of the 4-digit code numbers in ICD-O if the in-situ form of that neoplasm exists and is diagnosed.

During the field trials of ICD-O, the question was asked why the behavior code digits /0, /1, /2, /3, /6, /9, were not in consecutive numerical order. In other words, why were not the digits, 0, 1, 2, 3, 4, 5 and 6 used? The answer is that the behavior code numbers used in ICD-O are the same as the behavior code numbers used in MOTNAC and SNOP. Thus the behavior code numbers used for ICD-O and included as part of the morphology code numbers in Chapter II of ICD-9 maintain compatibility with many thousands of cases coded all over the world by SNOP and MOTNAC during the past ten years.

Cancer and carcinoma

The words "cancer" and "carcinoma" are often (incorrectly) used interchangeably; e.g., "Squamous cell cancer" is used for "Squamous cell carcinoma". To code the former as the latter would be reasonable. However, "Spindle cell cancer" could refer either to "Spindle cell sarcoma" or to "Spindle cell carcinoma". In ICD-O the word "cancer" is listed only once—as a synonym of the non-specific term "Malignant neoplasm" M-8000/3. Obviously, ICD-O cannot provide specific code numbers for all the instances in which the word "cancer" is used loosely and imprecisely as a part of a histologic diagnosis.

CODE FOR HISTOLOGIC GRADING AND DIFFERENTIATION

A one digit code number has been included in ICD-O to designate the grade or differentiation of malignant neoplasms as listed below:

Code No.

1.......... Grade I............. Well differentiated
                                  Differentiated

2.......... Grade II............Moderately differentiated
                                  Moderately well differentiated

3.......... Grade III...........Poorly differentiated

4.......... Grade IV ....Undifferentiated
                                  Anaplastic

9.......... Grade or differentiation not determined, not stated or
            not applicable

The code numbers for histologic grading and differentiation are independent of the 5-digit morphology and behavior code numbers which have been assigned to the terms listed in ICD-O and would be recorded in a different field from the morphology and behavior code numbers.

The use of grading varies greatly among pathologists throughout the world, and in many instances malignant tumors are not routinely graded. In the grading code listed above the code numbers 1 to 4 are used to designate grades I to IV respectively. Listed in a separate column are words used to designate degrees of differentiation. There is great variability in the use of these words by various pathologists. In general the adverbs, "well", "moderately" and "poorly", are used to indicate degrees of differentiation, which approximate grades I, II and III. "Undifferentiated" and "anaplastic" usually correspond to grade IV. Thus the diagnoses, "Squamous cell carcinoma, grade II" or "Moderately well differentiated squamous cell carcinoma", would both be coded to the morphology code number M-8070/3 and the grading (or differentiation) code number would be "2". In this example, the grading code "2" could be placed in a column immediately after the 5-digit morphology code number, so the full code number would be M-8070/32, or the "2" could be placed in a column separated from the morphology code number. It should be apparent from this example that the morphology code (M-8070/3) for "Squamous cell carcinoma" is the same whether the grading code is used or not. It is suggested that the higher number in the grading code should be used when diagnoses indicate two different degrees of grading or differentiation. Thus the statement "Moderately differentiated squamous cell carcinoma with poorly differentiated areas" should be given the grading code number "3". Its complete code number would therefore be M-8070/33.

The words used to designate degrees of differentiation—"well differentiated", "poorly differentiated", "anaplastic", etc.—have in a number of instances been used as an integral part of the histologic names for certain neoplasms. Thus "Well differentiated lymphocytic lymphoma" is an accepted histologic term and has been assigned the morphology code number 9620/3 in ICD-O. Obviously, a separate grading or differentiation code is not needed for this histologic diagnosis and, in fact, there is no problem if the coder does not use the grading code provided in ICD-O.

In addition to the malignant lymphomas, there are approximately 15 other histologic terms for neoplasms in ICD-O which are modified by words such as "anaplastic", "well differentiated", "undifferentiated", etc. Examples are: "Malignant teratoma, anaplastic type" (M-9082/3), "Retinoblastoma, differentiated type" (M-9511/3), and "Follicular adenocarcinoma, well differentiated type" (M-8331/3). To help obviate possible confusion, the word "type" has also been added to these terms to indicate that the modifying word is an integral part of the term used for the neoplasm.

For example, the histologic term "Anaplastic type carcinoma" has the code number M-8021/3 in ICD-O and this code number would also be used if the diagnosis were simply "anaplastic carcinoma". In other words, a grading code number is not necessary for this particular diagnosis. If, on the other hand, a grading code is used, the grading code number "4" would be used and the complete code number for this diagnosis would be M-8021/34. Obviously the grading code numbers can be applied to all the malignant neoplasms listed in ICD-O if the diagnosis includes information about grade or differentiation. For example, the grading code number "4" should be added to the morphology code number 8070/3 to code completely the diagnosis "Anaplastic squamous cell carcinoma", i.e., M-8070/34. It would be inaccurate to code this diagnosis to the morphology number 8021/3 for "Anaplastic type carcinoma". Furthermore, because the grading code in ICD-O is separate from and independent of the morphology and behavior code numbers, the grading code can also be used for metastases or for in-situ neoplasms. Thus the diagnosis of "Metastatic anaplastic squamous cell carcinoma" would be coded M-8070/64.

SITE-SPECIFIC MORPHOLOGY TERMS

Some terms for neoplasms are specific for certain sites or types of tissue. For example, "Nephroblastoma" (M-8960/3), by definition, always arises in the kidney; "Hepatocellular carcinoma" (M-8170/3) is always primary in the liver; "Basal cell carcinoma" (M-8090/3) usually arises in the skin and "Meningioma" (M-9530/0) in the meninges. To facilitate the coding of such terms, an appropriate topography number has been added to them in parentheses in both the numerical list of morphology and the alphabetic index. Thus, "Nephroblastoma" is followed by the topography number for kidney (T-189.0) and "Hepatocellular carcinoma" by the topography number for liver (T-155.0). In the case of "Basal cell carcinoma", the topography number for skin (T-173.__) is given with the fourth digit left open. The appropriate fourth digit for the site reported should be added; for example, a "Basal cell carcinoma of the face" would be given the site code T-173.3 (Skin of face) while one of the arm would be coded T-173.6 (Skin of arm). Similarly, the fourth digit is left open in the topography number (T-192.__) that follows "Meningioma" since the site involved may be either "Cerebral meninges" (T-192.1), "Spinal meninges" (T-192.3) or "Meninges, NOS" (T-192.1). In these examples, the T-numbers assigned to the morphologic terms should be used even if the topographic site is not given in the diagnosis. Site-specific T-numbers have not been assigned to many of the morphology terms because these histologic types of neoplasms can arise in more than one organ or topographic site. For example, "Adenocarcinoma, NOS" has no site-specific T-number because it can be primary in many different organs.

Occasionally a problem arises when a site is given in a diagnosis which is different from the site indicated by the site-specific T-number. In such instances, the site-specific T-number should be ignored and the appropriate T-number for the topography included in the diagnosis should be used. For example, the site-specific T-number, T-174.__ (Female breast) is added to the morphologic term "Infiltrating duct carcinoma", because this term is usually used for a type of carcinoma which arises in the breast. However, if the term "Infiltrating duct carcinoma" were used for a primary carcinoma arising in the pancreas, the correct T-number would be 157.9 (Pancreas, NOS).

It should be obvious that the T-numbers assigned to morphology terms designate the usual primary sites of origin of particular neoplasms and should not be used for coding the sites of metastases. An unlikely, but possible example would be the diagnosis "Hepatocellular carcinoma of the lung", for which the topography number for lung (T-162.9) should be used instead of T-155.0. In all probability, this diagnosis actually means that the hepatocellular carcinoma is metastatic in the lung, even though the word "metastatic" does not appear in the diagnosis. If this assumption is correct, the proper code numbers for that diagnosis would be T-162.9 (Lung) and M-8170/6 (Metastatic hepatocellular carcinoma).

PSEUDO-TOPOGRAPHIC MORPHOLOGY TERMS

Certain neoplasms have names that could be interpreted as implying a topographic location but these should not necessarily be coded to that site. For example, "Bile duct carcinoma" (M-8160/3) is a specific histologic type, usually found in the liver (T-155.0), and therefore should not be coded to the bile duct. "Sweat gland carcinoma" also has a specific morphology code number (M-8400/3).

Neoplasms of the minor salivary glands can be found anywhere in the oral cavity and neighboring organs and include several histologic types such as "Adenoid cystic carcinoma", "Malignant mixed tumor" and "Adenocarcinoma, NOS". Hence there is no distinctive morphologic code number for "Minor salivary gland carcinoma". Since all types of adenocarcinoma of the mouth or oral cavity are considered to be of minor salivary gland origin, the words "Minor salivary gland" should be ignored in a diagnosis such as "Minor salivary gland adenoid cystic carcinoma of the hard palate". In this example, the "Adenoid cystic carcinoma" (M-8200/3) should be coded to the topographic site, "Hard palate" (T-145.2). If no site of origin is given in a diagnosis such as "Minor salivary gland adenocarcinoma" the topography code number for oral cavity, T-145.9, which includes "Minor salivary gland, NOS" should be used.

COMPOUND MORPHOLOGIC DIAGNOSES

Some tumors have more than one histologic pattern. The most common combinations have been listed in ICD-O; e.g., "Mixed adenocarcinoma and squamous cell carcinoma" (M-8560/3), "Papillary and follicular adenocarcinoma" (M-8340/3), and "Mixed basal-squamous cell carcinoma" (M-8094/3).

The compound term "Fibromyxosarcoma" is listed in ICD-O with its code number M-8811/3. However, "Myxofibrosarcoma" does not appear in ICD-O. "Myxofibrosarcoma" is the same as "Fibromyxosarcoma", only the prefixes have been inverted, and therefore should also be coded M-8811/3. It was impossible to list all the combinations and permutations of such compound terms. The coder must check various permutations of the prefixes in these compound terms if the version sought is not listed in ICD-O.

Another type of coding difficulty arises if the diagnosis includes two modifying adjectives, which have different code numbers. An example is "Transitional cell epidermoid carcinoma". "Transitional cell carcinoma, NOS" is M-8120/3 and "Epidermoid carcinoma, NOS" is M-8070/3. The diagnostic phrase "Transitional cell epidermoid carcinoma" does not describe two different kinds of carcinoma, so coding to both numbers is incorrect. In such circumstances, use the higher number—M-8120/3 in this example—as it is usually more specific.

MULTIPLE NEOPLASMS

Multiple neoplasms in the same individual at the same time present many coding difficulties and specific solutions to all problems cannot be provided.

The following general rules are applicable:

1. Two or more separate neoplasms of different 3- or 4-digit sites should be coded separately, even though the morphologic type is the same for all. For example, "Squamous cell carcinoma of forehead and arm" should be coded twice: T-173.3 M-8070/3 (Squamous cell carcinoma of skin of forehead) and T-173.6 M-8070/3 (Squamous cell carcinoma of skin of arm). A more difficult example for coding multiple topographic sites is represented by the ambiguous diagnosis "Carcinoma of the adrenal gland and cecum". One cannot determine whether there are two separate carcinomas, one in the adrenal gland and one in the cecum, or whether

there is one carcinoma, which is primary in one or the other of these topographic sites with extension or metastases to the other topographic site. More exact information is needed before coding such a diagnosis.

2. Certain types of tumors occur in multiple sites; such diagnoses should be coded as a single neoplasm and the T-code chosen to include if possible, all the sites mentioned. For example, "Multiple polyposis in ascending and transverse colon" should be coded T-153.9 (Colon, NOS) and M-8221/0 (Multiple polyposis).

3. T-196.8 (Lymph nodes of multiple regions) is provided for coding the topography of certain neoplasms, chiefly malignant lymphomas which often involve multiple groups of lymph nodes. For example, T-196.8 might be used for "Malignant lymphoma, mixed cell type involving abdominal and inguinal lymph nodes". Alternatively these specific lymph nodes might be coded to the topography code numbers, T-196.2 and T-196.5. Many malignant lymphomas arise in other organs including stomach, intestine, tonsil, etc. and should be coded to these sites. For this reason, a site-specific T-number could not be assigned to the malignant lymphomas. However, if the diagnosis of any type of malignant lymphoma, e.g., "Hodgkin's disease" or "Lymphosarcoma, NOS" does not include a specific topographic site, use T-196.9 "Lymph node, NOS" or T-196.8 if multiple lymph nodes are involved.

4. Two or more separate neoplasms of different morphology should be coded separately, even though arising in the same site. For example, "Adenocarcinoma and Malignant carcinoid of transverse colon" should be coded T-153.1 M-8140/3 and T-153.1 M-8240/3. Similarly, a testis containing a "Seminoma and an Embryonal carcinoma" would be coded T-186.9 M-9061/3 and T-186.9 M-9070/3.

5. Multiple sites are often listed in diagnoses for a single neoplasm because the precise site of origin cannot be determined. A tumor that overlaps the boundaries of two or more subcategories of a 3-digit rubric and whose point of origin cannot be assigned to one of the 4-digit subcategories within that rubric should be assigned to ".8". For example, the diagnosis "Carcinoma of upper and middle thirds of esophagus" should be coded to 150.8. This diagnosis implies that there is a single carcinoma which has extended to involve two different parts of the esophagus. A few inclusive site codes have been provided in ICD-O and ICD-9. Examples are 149.8 (Neoplasms of lip, oral cavity and pharynx), 159.8 (Digestive organs and peritoneum), and 165.8 (Respiratory and intrathoracic organs). These inclusive site codes can be used for neoplasms, which overlap the boundaries of two or more 3-digit categories.

NO MICROSCOPIC CONFIRMATION OF TUMOR

A set of code numbers, M-9990/__, has been provided to record cases which have a clinical diagnosis of neoplasia or cancer but which have no microscopic confirmation or histologic diagnosis. These code numbers can be used when it is known that a tissue or cytologic specimen has not been examined microscopically and thus the neoplasm has not been classified histologically. Also a case may be clinically diagnosed as cancer even though a microscopic or cytologic examination was performed but was negative. The 5th digit in this set of code numbers should be selected in accordance with the clinical evaluation of the malignancy of the tumor. The listing of these code numbers appears in ICD-O as follows:

999 NO MICROSCOPIC CONFIRMATION
OF TUMOR

9990/0 No microscopic confirmation; clinically
benign tumor

9990/1 No microscopic confirmation; clinically
tumor, NOS

9990/3 No microscopic confirmation; clinically
malignant tumor *(cancer)*

9990/6 No microscopic confirmation; clinically
metastatic tumor *(cancer)*

ICD-O does not include a set of code numbers for various methods of diagnosis. Most tumor registries include such information in a separate field with appropriate code numbers designating the basis for the diagnosis, e.g., clinical or X-ray, microscopically proven from a surgical or biopsy specimen, autopsy, cytology, etc. The M-9990 code numbers in ICD-O do not provide for detailed coding of methods of diagnosis. If a separate "Method of diagnosis code" is used, the M-9990/__ code numbers in ICD-O can be ignored.

FUNCTION OF NEOPLASMS

ICD-O does not provide code numbers for the function of neoplasms; e.g., catecholamine production by a malignant pheochromocytoma (T-194.0 M-8700/3). Separate codes, such as those in Chapter III of ICD-9 can be used to record some of the types of functions of neoplasms; 255.6 in this example.

CYTOLOGY DIAGNOSES

ICD-O and ICD-9 are not structured to be used for cytology diagnoses. In other words, ICD-O topography does not specifically include 3- or 4-digit code numbers for sputum, vagino-cervical secretions or for fluids such as spinal fluid, urine, pleural effusion or ascitic fluid. If the topographic sites in ICD-O are used for cytology diagnoses, e.g., if "Pleura, NOS" (T-163.9) is used for pleural fluids, it is important to be able to identify and separate these coded cytology diagnoses from diagnoses based on tissue examinations. In most pathology departments the cytology diagnoses can be identified and separated from surgical pathology or autopsy diagnoses by the different types of accession numbers used for these various records. In a tumor registry, a method of diagnosis code may be used and will provide for this separation of coded data. The morphology section of ICD-O does not provide for coding such cytology findings as Papanicolaou class because these do not represent specific morphologic types of neoplasms.

TUMOR-LIKE LESIONS AND CONDITIONS

Diagnoses of certain non-neoplastic, tumor-like lesions and conditions are often recorded in cancer registries. Some of these are "tumor-like" or have names which can be confused with the names of neoplasms; others are of special interest because of their possible relationship to neoplasms. Most of them are included as tumor-like lesions in the WHO series on the *International Histological Classification of Tumours*. In ICD-O, these tumor-like lesions and conditions are listed in the alphabetic index without any morphology code numbers. Two examples of such listing are:

M------- Adenosis, sclerosing *(SNOMED M-74220)*

M------- Adenomatous goiter *(SNOMED M-71640)*

Code numbers appearing in parentheses after these terms are from the first edition of SNOMED[1], which has been developed as a revision and expansion of SNOP. A separate alphabetic list of the tumor-like lesions and conditions is included in ICD-O following the main alphabetic index.

FUTURE EDITIONS OF ICD-O

It is not planned to publish a second edition of ICD-O for several years, probably for at least 10 years when the Tenth Revision of ICD is expected to be published. In the interim, suggestions for additions or changes in this first edition of ICD-O should be sent to the World Health Organization, Geneva, Switzerland.

Preparations are being made for this first edition of ICD-O to be issued in other languages, including French, German, Italian, Japanese, Portuguese, Russian and Spanish.

---

[1]Systematized Nomenclature of Medicine, Chicago, Ill., College of American Pathologists (1976).

SUMMARY OF PRINCIPAL
RULES AND CONVENTIONS FOR USING ICD-O

In the interest of conformity in the use of ICD-O, the following rules and conventions are suggested:

1. Codes in ICD-O

A 10 digit field should be provided for coding topography (4 digits), morphology and behavior (5 digits) and grading or differentiation (1 digit). The complete code for the diagnosis "Moderately well differentiated squamous cell carcinoma of the base of tongue" is T-141.0 M-8070/32. See Introduction, page v.

2. Topographic regions and ill-defined sites

Ill-defined sites, such as "Ankle", have several component tissues. If the diagnosis does not specify the tissue of origin, use the appropriate tissue suggested in the alphabetic index for each ill-defined site in preference to the "NOS" category. For example, "Squamous cell carcinoma of the ankle" should be coded to T-173.7 (Skin of ankle) rather than T-195.5 (Ankle, NOS). See Introduction, page ix.

3. Prefixes

If a topographic site is modified by a prefix such as peri-, para-, etc. and is not specifically listed in ICD-O, code to the appropriate ill-defined subcategory. This is usually 195.__ unless the type of tumor indicates origin from a particular tissue. This general rule also applies to imprecise phrases such as "area of" or "region of". See Introduction, page x.

4. Tumors involving more than one topographic category or subcategory

A tumor that overlaps the boundaries of two or more categories or subcategories and whose point of origin cannot be determined, should be coded to subcategory ".8" when an appropriate ".8" subcategory is provided. See Introduction, page xix and Note, page 1.

5. Site-specific morphology terms

The appropriate T-numbers are listed in parentheses after those morphology terms which are site-specific; e.g., "Nephroblastoma" (T-189.0). If no site is indicated in the diagnosis, this T-number should be used. If a site is given, which is different from the site indicated by the T-number, ignore the T-number and code the appropriate T-number for the site in the diagnosis. Site-specific T-numbers should not be used for coding metastases.

Only 3-digit T-numbers are given for some sites, e.g., T-173.__ (skin) because the appropriate 4th digit cannot be assigned in advance. See Introduction, page $xvii$.

6. Topography sites for lymphomas

Lymphomas occur in specific organs, e.g., stomach, as well as in one or more lymph nodes and therefore are not assigned a site-specific T-number. If no site is indicated, code to T-196.9 (Lymph node, NOS) or, if multiple nodes are involved, code to T-196.8. See Introduction, page *xix*.

7. Compound morphologic diagnoses

Not all forms of compound words are listed. For example, "Fibromyxosarcoma" is in ICD-O but "Myxofibrosarcoma" is not. The coder must check various permutations of the prefixes if the first one is not found. See Introduction, page *xviii*.

If a term has two or more modifying adjectives, which have different code numbers, code to the one with the highest code number, as it is usually more specific. See Introduction, page *xviii*.

8. Multiple neoplasms

Multiple neoplasms present many coding difficulties: (1) two or more separate neoplasms in different topographic sites; (2) certain conditions, which are characterized by multiple tumors; (3) lymphomas, which often involve multiple lymph nodes or organs at diagnosis; (4) two or more neoplasms of different morphology arising in the same site; and, (5) a single neoplasm involving multiple sites whose precise origin cannot be determined. See general rules for these problems, Introduction, page *xviii*.

9. Behavior code in morphology

The use of the 5th digit behavior code numbers is explained in the Introduction, page *xii*, and in Table 1, page *xiv*. The appropriate 5th digit code should be used even though the exact term is not listed in ICD-O; e.g., "Benign chordoma" as a diagnosis should be coded M-9370/0.

10. Grading or differentiation code

If a diagnosis indicates two different degrees of grade or differentiation (e.g., "well and poorly differentiated" or "grades II-III"), code to the higher grade code. See Introduction, page *xvi*.

TOPOGRAPHY

NUMERICAL LIST

Note: *In categories T-140 to T-199, neoplasms should be assigned to the sub-category that includes the point of origin of the tumor. Tumors that overlap the boundaries of two or more sub-categories and whose point of origin cannot be determined should be classified to sub-category ".8". For example, a neoplasm of cervico-thoracic esophagus should be assigned to T-150.8 .*

140-149 LIP, ORAL CAVITY AND PHARYNX

140 LIP *(excludes Skin of lip T-173.0)*

140.0 Upper lip, NOS *(excludes Skin of upper lip T-173.0)*
External upper lip
Vermilion border of upper lip

140.1 Lower lip, NOS *(excludes Skin of lower lip T-173.0)*
External lower lip
Vermilion border of lower lip

140.3 Mucosa of upper lip
Inner aspect of upper lip
Frenulum of upper lip

140.4 Mucosa of lower lip
Inner aspect of lower lip
Frenulum of lower lip

140.5 Mucosa of lip, NOS
Inner aspect of lip, NOS
Internal lip, NOS
Frenulum of lip, NOS
Frenulum labii, NOS

140.6 Commissure of lip
Labial commissure

140.8 *(See note page 1)*

140.9 Lip, NOS *(excludes Skin of lip T-173.0)*
External lip, NOS
Vermilion border of lip, NOS

141 TONGUE

141.0 Base of tongue, NOS
Dorsal surface of base of tongue
Posterior third of tongue
Posterior tongue, NOS
Root of tongue

141.1 Dorsal surface of tongue, NOS
Anterior 2/3 of tongue, dorsal surface
Midline of tongue
Dorsal surface of anterior tongue

141.2 Border of tongue
Tip of tongue

141.3 Ventral surface of tongue, NOS
Anterior 2/3 of tongue, ventral surface
Frenulum linguae
Ventral surface of anterior tongue

141.4 Anterior 2/3 of tongue, NOS
Anterior tongue, NOS

141.5 Junctional zone of tongue

141.6 Lingual tonsil

141.8 *(See note page 1)*

141.9 Tongue, NOS
Lingual, NOS

142 MAJOR SALIVARY GLANDS

Note: *Neoplasms of minor salivary glands should be classified according to their anatomical site; if location is not specified, classify to T-145.9.*

142.0 Parotid gland
    Parotid, NOS
Stensen's duct
    Parotid gland duct

142.1 Submandibular gland
    Submaxillary gland
Wharton's duct
    Submaxillary gland duct

142.2 Sublingual gland
    Sublingual gland duct

142.8 *(See note page 1)*

142.9 Major salivary gland, NOS
    Salivary gland, NOS *(excludes Minor salivary gland, NOS T-145.9; see Introduction, page xviii and note under T-142)*

143 GUM

143.0 Upper gum
    Maxillary gingiva
    Upper alveolar mucosa
    Upper alveolar ridge mucosa
    Upper alveolus
    Upper gingiva

143.1 Lower gum
    Mandibular gingiva
    Lower alveolar mucosa
    Lower alveolar ridge mucosa
    Lower alveolus
    Lower gingiva

143.8 *(See note page 1)*

143.9 Gum, NOS
    Gingiva, NOS
    Alveolar mucosa, NOS
    Alveolar ridge mucosa, NOS
    Alveolus, NOS
Periodontal tissue
Tooth socket

144 FLOOR OF MOUTH

144.0 Anterior floor of mouth

144.1 Lateral floor of mouth

144.8 *(See note page 1)*

144.9 Floor of mouth, NOS

145 OTHER AND UNSPECIFIED PARTS OF MOUTH

145.0 Cheek mucosa
    Buccal mucosa
    Internal cheek

145.1 Vestibule of mouth
    Alveolar sulcus
    Buccal sulcus
    Labial sulcus

145.2 Hard palate

145.3 Soft palate, NOS *(excludes Nasopharyngeal surface of soft palate T-147.3)*

145.4 Uvula

145.5 Palate, NOS
    Roof of mouth
    Junction of hard and soft palate

145.6 Retromolar area
    Retromolar triangle
    Retromolar trigone

145.8 *(See note page 1)*

145.9 Oral cavity
    Buccal cavity
    Mouth, NOS
    Oral mucosa
    Minor salivary gland, NOS *(See Introduction page xviii and note under T-142)*

146 OROPHARYNX

146.0 Tonsil, NOS *(excludes Lingual tonsil T-141.6 and Pharyngeal tonsil T-147.1)*
Faucial tonsil
Palatine tonsil

146.1 Tonsillar fossa

146.2 Tonsillar pillar
Faucial pillar
Glossopalatine fold

146.3 Vallecula epiglottica
Vallecula, NOS

146.4 Anterior surface of epiglottis

146.5 Junctional region of oropharynx

146.6 Lateral wall of oropharynx
Lateral wall of mesopharynx

146.7 Posterior wall of oropharynx
Posterior wall of mesopharynx

146.8 Other parts of oropharynx
Branchial cleft *(site of neoplasm)*
(See also note page 1)

146.9 Oropharynx, NOS
Mesopharynx, NOS
Fauces, NOS

147 NASOPHARYNX

147.0 Superior wall of nasopharynx
Roof of nasopharynx

147.1 Posterior wall of nasopharynx
Adenoid
Pharyngeal tonsil

147.2 Lateral wall of nasopharynx
Fossa of Rosenmüller

147.3 Anterior wall of nasopharynx
Nasopharyngeal surface of soft palate
Pharyngeal fornix
Choana
Posterior margin of nasal septum

147.8 *(See note page 1)*

147.9 Nasopharynx, NOS
Nasopharyngeal wall

148 HYPOPHARYNX

148.0 Postcricoid region
Cricopharynx
Cricoid, NOS

148.1 Pyriform sinus
Pyriform fossa

148.2 Aryepiglottic fold, NOS *(excludes Laryngeal aspect of aryepiglottic fold T-161.1)*
Hypopharyngeal aspect of aryepiglottic fold
Arytenoid fold

148.3 Posterior wall of hypopharynx

148.8 *(See note page 1)*

148.9 Hypopharynx, NOS
Laryngopharynx
Hypopharyngeal wall

149 PHARYNX AND ILL-DEFINED SITES IN LIP, ORAL CAVITY AND PHARYNX

149.0 Pharynx, NOS
Pharyngeal wall, NOS
Wall of pharynx, NOS
Lateral wall of pharynx, NOS
Posterior wall of pharynx, NOS
Retropharynx
Throat

149.1 Waldeyer's ring, NOS

149.8 Note: *Neoplasms of lip, oral cavity and pharynx whose point of origin cannot be assigned to any one of the categories T-140 to T-148.*

149.9 Ill-defined sites in lip, oral cavity and pharynx

150-159 DIGESTIVE ORGANS AND PERITONEUM

150 ESOPHAGUS

150.0 Cervical esophagus

150.1 Thoracic esophagus

150.2 Abdominal esophagus

150.3 Upper third of esophagus
 Proximal third of esophagus

150.4 Middle third of esophagus

150.5 Lower third of esophagus
 Distal third of esophagus

150.8 *(See note page 1)*

150.9 Esophagus, NOS

151 STOMACH

151.0 Cardia, NOS
 Gastric cardia
 Cardio-esophageal junction
 Esophagogastric junction
 Gastroesophageal junction

151.1 Pylorus
 Pyloric canal
 Prepylorus

151.2 Pyloric antrum
 Antrum of stomach
 Gastric antrum

151.3 Fundus of stomach
 Gastric fundus

151.4 Body of stomach
 Corpus of stomach
 Gastric corpus

151.5 Lesser curvature of stomach, NOS *(not classifiable to T-151.1 to T-151.4)*

151.6 Greater curvature of stomach, NOS *(not classifiable to T-151.0 to T-151.4)*

151.8 Other parts of stomach
 Anterior wall of stomach, NOS *(not classifiable to T-151.0 to T-151.4)*
 Posterior wall of stomach, NOS *(not classifiable to T-151.0 to T-151.4)*
 (See also note page 1)

151.9 Stomach, NOS
 Gastric, NOS

152 SMALL INTESTINE

152.0 Duodenum

152.1 Jejunum

152.2 Ileum *(excludes Ileocecal valve T-153.4)*

152.3 Meckel's diverticulum *(site of neoplasm)*

152.8 *(See note page 1)*

152.9 Small intestine
 Small bowel

153 COLON

153.0 Hepatic flexure of colon

153.1 Transverse colon

153.2 Descending colon
 Left colon

153.3 Sigmoid colon
 Sigmoid, NOS
 Sigmoid flexure of colon
 Pelvic colon

153.4 Cecum
 Ileocecal valve
 Ileocecal junction

153.5 Appendix

153.6 Ascending colon
    Right colon

153.7 Splenic flexure of colon

153.8 *(See note page 1)*

153.9 Colon, NOS
    Large intestine *(excludes Rectum, NOS*
    T-154.1 and Rectosigmoid junction
    T-154.0)
    Large bowel

154 RECTUM, RECTOSIGMOID JUNCTION, ANAL CANAL AND ANUS, NOS

154.0 Rectosigmoid junction
    Rectosigmoid, NOS
    Rectosigmoid colon
    Colon and rectum
    Pelvi-rectal junction

154.1 Rectum, NOS
    Rectal ampulla

154.2 Anal canal
    Anal sphincter

154.3 Anus, NOS *(excludes Skin of anus and*
    Perianal skin T-173.5)

154.8 Other parts of rectum
    Anorectal junction
    Anorectum
    Cloacogenic zone
    (See also note page 1)

155 LIVER AND INTRAHEPATIC BILE DUCTS

155.0 Liver
    Hepatic, NOS

155.1 Intrahepatic bile duct
    Biliary canaliculus
    Cholangiole

156 GALLBLADDER AND EXTRAHEPATIC BILE DUCTS

156.0 Gallbladder

156.1 Extrahepatic bile duct
    Bile duct, NOS
      Biliary duct, NOS
    Choledochal duct
    Common bile duct
      Common duct
    Cystic bile duct
      Cystic duct
    Hepatic bile duct
      Hepatic duct
    Sphincter of Oddi

156.2 Ampulla of Vater
    Periampullary

156.8 *(See note page 1)*

156.9 Biliary tract, NOS

157 PANCREAS

157.0 Head of pancreas

157.1 Body of pancreas

157.2 Tail of pancreas

157.3 Pancreatic duct
    Duct of Santorini
    Duct of Wirsung

157.4 Islets of Langerhans
    Islands of Langerhans

157.8 *(See note page 1)*

157.9 Pancreas, NOS

158 RETROPERITONEUM AND PERITONEUM

158.0 Retroperitoneum
Periadrenal tissue
Perinephric tissue
Peripancreatic tissue
Perirenal tissue
Retrocecal tissue
Retroperitoneal tissue

158.8 Specified parts of peritoneum
Mesentery
Mesoappendix
Mesocolon
Omentum
Pelvic peritoneum
Rectouterine pouch
Cul de sac
Pouch of Douglas
(See also note page 1)

158.9 Peritoneum, NOS
Peritoneal cavity

159 OTHER AND ILL-DEFINED SITES WITHIN DIGESTIVE ORGANS AND PERITONEUM

159.0 Intestinal tract, NOS
Bowel, NOS
Intestine, NOS

159.8 Note: *Neoplasms of digestive organs and peritoneum whose point of origin cannot be assigned to any one of the categories T-150 to T-158.*

159.9 Gastrointestinal tract, NOS
Alimentary tract, NOS
Digestive organs, NOS

160-165 RESPIRATORY SYSTEM AND INTRATHORACIC ORGANS

160 NASAL CAVITIES, ACCESSORY SINUSES, MIDDLE EAR AND INNER EAR

160.0 Nasal cavity *(excludes Nose, NOS T-195.0)*
Internal nose
Naris
Nasal cartilage
Nasal mucosa
Nasal septum, NOS *(excludes Posterior margin of nasal septum T-147.3)*
Nasal turbinate
Nostril
Vestibule of nose

160.1 Middle ear
Inner ear
Auditory tube
Eustachian tube
Mastoid antrum
Tympanic cavity

160.2 Maxillary sinus
Maxillary antrum
Antrum, NOS

160.3 Ethmoid sinus

160.4 Frontal sinus

160.5 Sphenoid sinus

160.8 *(See note page 1)*

160.9 Accessory sinus, NOS
Accessory nasal sinus
Paranasal sinus

161 LARYNX

161.0 Glottis
Intrinsic larynx
Laryngeal commissure
Vocal cord, NOS
True vocal cord
True cord

161.1 Supraglottis
Epiglottis, NOS *(excludes Anterior surface of epiglottis T-146.4)*
Extrinsic larynx
Laryngeal aspect of aryepiglottic fold
Posterior surface of epiglottis
Ventricular band of larynx
    False vocal cord
    False cord

161.2 Subglottis

161.3 Laryngeal cartilage
Arytenoid cartilage
Cricoid cartilage
Cuneiform cartilage
Thyroid cartilage

161.8 *(See note page 1)*

161.9 Larynx, NOS

162 TRACHEA, BRONCHUS, AND LUNG

162.0 Trachea

162.2 Main bronchus
Carina
Hilus of lung

162.3 Upper lobe, lung
Lingula of lung
Upper lobe, bronchus

162.4 Middle lobe, lung
Middle lobe, bronchus

162.5 Lower lobe, lung
Lower lobe, bronchus

162.8 Other parts of lung or bronchus
(See also note page 1)

162.9 Lung, NOS
Bronchus, NOS
Bronchiole
Bronchogenic
Pulmonary, NOS

163 PLEURA

163.0 Parietal pleura

163.1 Visceral pleura

163.8 *(See note page 1)*

163.9 Pleura, NOS

164 THYMUS, HEART AND MEDIASTINUM

164.0 Thymus

164.1 Heart
Endocardium
Epicardium
Myocardium
Pericardium
Cardiac ventricle
Cardiac atrium

164.2 Anterior mediastinum

164.3 Posterior mediastinum

164.8 *(See note page 1)*

164.9 Mediastinum, NOS

165 OTHER AND ILL-DEFINED SITES WITHIN RESPIRATORY SYSTEM AND INTRATHORACIC ORGANS

165.0 Upper respiratory tract

165.8 Note: *Neoplasms of respiratory and intrathoracic organs whose point of origin cannot be assigned to any one of the categories T-160 to T-164.*

165.9 Ill-defined sites within respiratory system
Respiratory tract, NOS

169 HEMATOPOIETIC AND RETICULOENDOTHELIAL SYSTEMS

169.0 Blood

169.1 Bone marrow

169.2 Spleen

169.3 Reticuloendothelial system, NOS

169.9 Hematopoietic system, NOS

170 BONES, JOINTS AND ARTICULAR CARTILAGE

170.0 Bones of skull and face and associated joints
(excludes Mandible T-170.1)
Calvarium
Cranial bone
Ethmoid bone
Facial bone
Frontal bone
Hyoid bone
Maxilla
   Upper jaw bone
Nasal bone
Occipital bone
Orbital bone
Parietal bone
Skull, NOS
Sphenoid bone
Temporal bone
Zygomatic bone

170.1 Mandible
   Jaw bone, NOS
     Lower jaw bone
Temporomandibular joint

170.2 Vertebral column *(excludes Sacrum and Coccyx T-170.6)*
Atlas
Axis
Bone of back
Intervertebral disc
Nucleus pulposus
Spinal column
Spine
Vertebra

170.3 Rib, Sternum, Clavicle and associated joints
Costal cartilage
Costovertebral joint
Sternocostal joint

170.4 Long bones of upper limb, scapula and associated joints
Acromioclavicular joint
Bone of arm
Bone of forearm
Bone of shoulder
Elbow joint
Humerus
Radius
Scapula
Shoulder girdle
Shoulder joint
Ulna

170.5 Short bones of upper limb and associated joints
Bone of finger
Bone of hand
Bone of thumb
Bone of wrist
Carpal bone
Hand joint
Metacarpal bone
Phalanx of hand
Wrist joint

170.6 Pelvic bones, Sacrum, Coccyx and associated joints
Acetabulum
Bone of hip
Coccyx
Hip joint
Ilium
Innominate bone
Ischium
Pelvic bone
Pubic bone
Sacrum
Symphysis pubis

170.7 Long bones of lower limb and associated joints

Bone of leg
Femur
Fibula
Knee joint, NOS
Semilunar cartilage
    Lateral meniscus of knee joint
    Medial meniscus of knee joint
Tibia

170.8 Short bones of lower limb and associated joints

Ankle joint
Bone of ankle
Bone of foot
Bone of heel
Bone of toe
Foot joint
Metatarsal bone
Patella
Phalanx of foot
Tarsal bone

170.9 Bone, NOS

Cartilage, NOS
Joint, NOS
Skeletal bone
Articular cartilage, NOS

171 CONNECTIVE, SUBCUTANEOUS AND OTHER SOFT TISSUES (includes Adipose tissue, Aponeuroses, Artery, Autonomic nervous system, Blood vessel, Bursa, Connective tissue, Fascia, Fatty tissue, Fibrous tissue, Ganglia, Ligament, Lymphatic, Muscle, Nerve, Parasympathetic nervous system, Peripheral nerve, Skeletal muscle, Spinal nerve, Subcutaneous tissue, Sympathetic nervous system, Synovia, Tendon, Tendon sheath, Vein, Vessel)

171.0 Connective, Subcutaneous and other Soft tissues of head, face, and neck
(excludes Connective tissue of orbit T-190.1 and Nasal cartilage T-160.0)

171.0 *(Cont'd)*

Connective, Subcutaneous and other Soft tissues *(see list under T-171)* of
cheek
chin
face
forehead
head
neck
scalp
temple
cervical region
pterygoid fossa
supraclavicular region

Auricular cartilage
    Cartilage of ear
Carotid artery
Cervical plexus
Masseter muscle
Pterygoid fossa, NOS
Sternocleidomastoid muscle

171.2 Connective, Subcutaneous and other Soft tissues of upper limb and shoulder

Connective, Subcutaneous and other Soft tissues *(see list under T-171)* of
antecubital space
arm
elbow
finger
forearm
hand
shoulder
thumb
wrist

Biceps brachii muscle
Brachialis muscle
Brachial nerve
Brachial plexus
Coracobrachialis muscle
Deltoideus muscle
Median nerve
Palmar aponeurosis
Palmar fascia
Radial artery
Radial nerve
Triceps brachii muscle
Ulnar artery
Ulnar nerve

171.3 Connective, Subcutaneous and other Soft tissues of lower limb and hip

Connective, Subcutaneous and other Soft tissues *(see list under T-171)* of
- ankle
- calf
- foot
- heel
- hip
- knee
- leg
- popliteal space
- thigh
- toe

Biceps femoris muscle
Femoral artery
Femoral nerve
Gastrocnemius muscle
Obturator nerve
Plantar aponeurosis
Plantar fascia
Quadriceps femoris muscle
Sciatic nerve

171.4 Connective, Subcutaneous and other Soft tissues of thorax *(excludes Thymus, Heart and Mediastinum T-164.__)*

Connective, Subcutaneous and other Soft tissues *(see list under T-171)* of
- axilla
- chest
- chest wall
- thoracic wall
- infraclavicular region
- scapular region

Aorta, NOS
Axillary artery
Diaphragm
Intercostal muscle
Intercostal nerve
Internal mammary artery
Latissimus dorsi muscle
Pectoralis major muscle
Subclavian artery
Superior vena cava
Thoracic duct
Trapezius muscle

171.5 Connective, Subcutaneous and other Soft tissues of abdomen

Connective, Subcutaneous and other Soft tissues *(see list under T-171)* of
- abdominal wall
- umbilicus

Abdominal aorta
Abdominal vena cava
Abdominal wall muscle
Celiac artery
Iliopsoas muscle
Inferior vena cava
Mesenteric artery
Psoas muscle
Rectus abdominis muscle
Renal artery
Vena cava, NOS

171.6 Connective, Subcutaneous and other Soft tissues of pelvis

Connective, Subcutaneous and other Soft tissues *(see list under T-171)* of
- buttock
- groin
- perineum
- gluteal region
- inguinal region
- sacrococcygeal region

Gluteus maximus muscle
Iliac artery
Iliac vein
Lumbosacral plexus
Sacral nerve
Sacral plexus

171.7 Connective, Subcutaneous and other Soft tissues of trunk

Connective, Subcutaneous and other Soft tissues *(see list under T-171)* of
- back
- flank
- trunk

Lumbar nerve

171.8 *(See note page 1)*

171.9 Connective, Subcutaneous and other Soft tissues, NOS

Adipose tissue, NOS
Aponeurosis, NOS
Artery, NOS
Autonomic nervous system
Blood vessel, NOS
Bursa, NOS
Connective tissue, NOS
Fascia, NOS
Fatty tissue, NOS
Fibrous tissue, NOS
Ganglia, NOS
Ligament, NOS
Lymphatic, NOS
Muscle, NOS
Nerve, NOS
Parasympathetic nervous system
Peripheral nerve, NOS
Skeletal muscle, NOS
Spinal nerve, NOS
Subcutaneous tissue, NOS
Sympathetic nervous system
Synovia, NOS
Tendon, NOS
Tendon sheath, NOS
Vein, NOS
Vessel, NOS

173 SKIN *(excludes Skin of labia majora T-184.1, Skin of vulva T-184.4, Skin of penis T-187.4 and Skin of scrotum T-187.7)*

173.0 Skin of lip, NOS
Skin of lower lip
Skin of upper lip

173.1 Eyelid
Lid, NOS
Palpebra
Canthus, NOS
Inner canthus
Lower lid
Meibomian gland
Outer canthus
Upper lid

173.2 External ear
Auricle, NOS
Pinna
Ceruminal gland
Concha
Ear, NOS
Ear lobule
Earlobe
External auditory canal
Auditory canal, NOS
Auricular canal, NOS
External auricular canal
Ear canal
External auditory meatus
Helix
Skin of auricle
Skin of ear
Tragus

173.3 Skin of other and unspecified parts of face

Skin of { cheek chin face forehead jaw nose temple

Ala nasi
Chin, NOS
Columnella
Eyebrow
Brow
External cheek
External nose
Forehead, NOS
Temple, NOS

173.4 Skin of scalp and neck
Skin of head, NOS
Skin of neck
Skin of scalp
Scalp, NOS
Skin of cervical region
Skin of supraclavicular region

173.5 Skin of trunk

Skin of
- abdomen
- abdominal wall
- anus
- axilla
- back
- breast
- buttock
- chest
- chest wall
- flank
- groin
- perineum
- thoracic wall
- thorax
- trunk
- umbilicus
- gluteal region
- infraclavicular region
- inguinal region
- sacrococcygeal region
- scapular region

Perianal skin
Umbilicus, NOS

173.6 Skin of arm and shoulder

Skin of
- antecubital space
- arm
- elbow
- finger
- forearm
- hand
- palm
- shoulder
- thumb
- upper limb
- wrist

Finger nail
Palmar skin

173.7 Skin of leg and hip

Skin of
- ankle
- calf
- foot
- heel
- hip
- knee
- leg
- lower limb
- popliteal space
- thigh
- toe

Plantar skin
Sole of foot
Toe nail

173.8 *(See note page 1)*

173.9 Skin, NOS *(excludes Skin of labia majora T-184.1, Skin of vulva T-184.4, Skin of penis T-187.4 and Skin of scrotum T-187.7)*

174 FEMALE BREAST *(excludes Skin of breast T-173.5)*

174.0 Nipple
Areola

174.1 Central portion of breast

174.2 Upper-inner quadrant of breast

174.3 Lower-inner quadrant of breast

174.4 Upper-outer quadrant of breast

174.5 Lower-outer quadrant of breast

174.6 Axillary tail of breast
Tail of breast

174.8 Inner breast
Lower breast
Midline of breast
Outer breast
Upper breast
(See also note page 1)

174.9 Female Breast, NOS *(excludes Skin of breast T- 173.5)*
 Breast, NOS *(excludes Skin of the breast T-173.5)*
 Mammary gland

175 MALE BREAST *(excludes Skin of breast T-173.5)*

175.9 Male breast, NOS *(excludes Skin of breast T-173.5)*

179-189 GENITOURINARY ORGANS

179 UTERUS, NOS

179.9 Uterus, NOS
 Uterine, NOS

180 CERVIX UTERI

180.0 Endocervix
 Internal os
 Cervical canal
 Endocervical canal
 Endocervical gland
 Nabothian gland

180.1 Exocervix
 External os

180.8 Other parts of cervix
 Cervical stump
 Squamocolumnar junction of cervix
 (See also note page 1)

180.9 Cervix uteri
 Cervix, NOS
 Uterine cervix

181 PLACENTA

181.9 Placenta
 Fetal membranes

182 CORPUS UTERI

182.0 Corpus uteri
 Body of uterus
 Endometrial gland
 Endometrial stroma
 Endometrium
 Fundus uteri
 Myometrium

182.1 Isthmus uteri
 Lower uterine segment

182.8 *(See note page 1)*

183 OVARY, FALLOPIAN TUBE AND BROAD LIGAMENT

183.0 Ovary

183.2 Fallopian tube
 Uterine tube

183.3 Broad ligament
 Mesovarium
 Parovarian region

183.4 Parametrium
 Uterine ligament
 Uterosacral ligament

183.5 Round ligament

183.8 Other parts of uterine adnexa
 Tubo-ovarian
 Utero-ovarian
 (See also note page 1)

183.9 Uterine adnexa
 Adnexa, NOS

184 OTHER AND UNSPECIFIED FEMALE GENITAL ORGANS

184.0 Vagina, NOS
Vaginal vault
Fornix of vagina
Gartner's duct
Hymen

184.1 Labium majus
Labia majora, NOS
Bartholin's gland
Skin of labia majora

184.2 Labium minus
Labia minora

184.3 Clitoris

184.4 Vulva, NOS
External female genitalia
Fourchette
Labium, NOS
  Labia, NOS
Mons pubis
Mons veneris
Pudendum
Skin of vulva

184.8 *(See note page 1)*

184.9 Female genital tract, NOS
Female genital organs, NOS
Female genitourinary tract, NOS
Urethrovaginal septum
Vesicocervical tissue
Vesicovaginal septum

185 PROSTATE GLAND

185.9 Prostate gland
Prostate, NOS

186 TESTIS

186.0 Undescended testis *(site of neoplasm)*
Retained testis *(site of neoplasm)*
Ectopic testis *(site of neoplasm)*

186.9 Testis, NOS
Descended testis
Scrotal testis
Testicle, NOS

187 PENIS AND OTHER MALE GENITAL ORGANS

187.1 Prepuce
Foreskin

187.2 Glans penis

187.3 Body of penis
Corpus cavernosum
Corpus of penis

187.4 Penis, NOS
Skin of penis

187.5 Epididymis

187.6 Spermatic cord
Vas deferens

187.7 Scrotum, NOS
Skin of scrotum

187.8 Other parts of male genital organs
Seminal vesicle
Tunica vaginalis
(See also note page 1)

187.9 Male genital organs, NOS
Male genital tract, NOS
Male genitourinary tract, NOS

188 URINARY BLADDER

188.0 Trigone of urinary bladder

188.1 Dome of urinary bladder

188.2 Lateral wall of urinary bladder

188.3 Anterior wall of urinary bladder

188.4 Posterior wall of urinary bladder

188.5 Bladder neck
Internal urethral orifice

188.6 Ureteric orifice

188.7 Urachus

188.8 *(See note page 1)*

188.9 Urinary bladder, NOS
Bladder, NOS
Bladder wall, NOS

189 KIDNEY AND OTHER URINARY ORGANS

189.0 Kidney, NOS
Renal, NOS
Kidney parenchyma

189.1 Renal pelvis
Pelvis of kidney
Renal calyces
Renal calyx
Pelvi-ureteric junction

189.2 Ureter

189.3 Urethra
Cowper's gland
Prostatic utricle
Urethral gland

189.4 Paraurethral gland

189.8 *(See note page 1)*

189.9 Urinary system, NOS

190 EYE AND LACRIMAL GLAND

190.0 Eyeball
Ciliary body
Crystalline lens
Iris
Sclera
Uveal tract
Intraocular

190.1 Orbit, NOS
Connective tissue of orbit
Extra-ocular muscle
Retrobulbar tissue
Soft tissue of orbit

190.2 Lacrimal gland

190.3 Conjunctiva

190.4 Cornea, NOS
Limbus of cornea

190.5 Retina

190.6 Choroid

190.7 Lacrimal duct, NOS
Nasal lacrimal duct
Nasolacrimal duct
Lacrimal sac

190.8 *(See note page 1)*

190.9 Eye, NOS

191-192 NERVOUS SYSTEM

191 BRAIN

191.0 Cerebrum
Basal ganglia
Central white matter
Cerebral cortex
Cerebral hemisphere
Cerebral white matter
Corpus striatum
Globus pallidus
Hypothalamus
Insula
Internal capsule
Island of Reil
Operculum
Pallium
Putamen
Rhinencephalon
Thalamus

191.1 Frontal lobe
Frontal pole

191.2 Temporal lobe
Hippocampus
Uncus

191.3 Parietal lobe

191.4 Occipital lobe
Occipital pole

191.5 Ventricle, NOS
Cerebral ventricle
Choroid plexus
Ependyma
Fourth ventricle
Lateral ventricle
Third ventricle

191.6 Cerebellum, NOS
Cerebellopontine angle
Vermis of cerebellum

191.7 Brain stem
Cerebral peduncle
Basis pedunculi
Medulla oblongata
Midbrain
Olive
Pons
Pyramid

191.8 Other parts of brain
Corpus callosum
Tapetum
(See also note page 1)

191.9 Brain, NOS
Intracranial site
Cranial fossa, NOS
Anterior cranial fossa
Middle cranial fossa
Posterior cranial fossa
Suprasellar

192 OTHER AND UNSPECIFIED PARTS OF NERVOUS SYSTEM
(excludes Peripheral nerves, Sympathetic and parasympathetic nerves and ganglia T-171.9)

192.0 Cranial nerve
Abducens nerve
Accessory nerve, NOS
Spinal accessory nerve
Acoustic nerve
Facial nerve
Glossopharyngeal nerve
Hypoglossal nerve
Oculomotor nerve
Olfactory nerve
Optic chiasm
Optic nerve
Optic tract
Trigeminal nerve
Trochlear nerve
Vagus nerve

192.1 Cerebral meninges
Arachnoid, NOS
Cranial dura mater
Cranial meninges
Cranial pia mater
Dura, NOS
Dura mater, NOS
Falx, NOS
Falx cerebelli
Falx cerebri
Intracranial arachnoid
Intracranial meninges
Meninges, NOS
Pia mater, NOS
Tentorium cerebelli
Tentorium, NOS

192.2 Spinal cord
Cauda equina
Cervical cord
Conus medullaris
Filum terminale
Lumbar cord
Sacral cord
Thoracic cord

192.3 Spinal meninges
Spinal arachnoid
Spinal dura mater
Spinal pia mater

192.8 *(See note page 1)*

192.9 Nervous system, NOS
Central nervous system
Epidural
Extradural
Parasellar

193-194 ENDOCRINE GLANDS

193 THYROID GLAND

193.9 Thyroid gland
Thyroid, NOS
Thyroglossal duct

194 OTHER ENDOCRINE GLANDS

194.0 Suprarenal gland
Adrenal gland
Adrenal, NOS
Adrenal cortex
Adrenal medulla

194.1 Parathyroid gland

194.3 Pituitary gland
Pituitary, NOS
Hypophysis
Craniopharyngeal duct
Rathke's pouch
Sella turcica
Pituitary fossa

194.4 Pineal gland

194.5 Carotid body

194.6 Aortic body and other paraganglia
Coccygeal body
Coccygeal glomus
Glomus jugulare
Para-aortic body
Organ of Zuckerkandl
Paraganglion

194.8 Multiple endocrine glands
Pluriglandular
(See also note page 1)

194.9 Endocrine gland, NOS

195 OTHER ILL-DEFINED SITES

195.0 Head, face or neck, NOS
Cheek, NOS
Jaw, NOS
Nose, NOS
Cervical region, NOS
Supraclavicular region, NOS

195.1 Thorax, NOS
Axilla, NOS
Chest, NOS
Chest wall, NOS
Intrathoracic site, NOS
Thoracic wall, NOS
Infraclavicular region, NOS
Scapular region, NOS

195.2 Abdomen, NOS
Abdominal wall, NOS
Intra-abdominal site, NOS

195.3 Pelvis, NOS
Buttock, NOS
Groin, NOS
Ischiorectal fossa
Pelvic wall, NOS
Perineum, NOS
Rectovaginal septum
Rectovesical septum
Gluteal region, NOS
Inguinal region, NOS
Perirectal region, NOS
Presacral region, NOS
Sacrococcygeal region, NOS

195.4 Upper limb, NOS
Antecubital space, NOS
Arm, NOS
Elbow, NOS
Finger, NOS
Forearm, NOS
Hand, NOS
Shoulder, NOS
Thumb, NOS
Wrist, NOS

195.5 Lower limb, NOS
Ankle, NOS
Calf, NOS
Foot, NOS
Heel, NOS
Hip, NOS
Knee, NOS
Leg, NOS
Popliteal space, NOS
Thigh, NOS
Toe, NOS

195.8 Other ill-defined sites
Back, NOS
Flank, NOS
Trunk, NOS

196 LYMPH NODES

196.0 Lymph nodes of head, face and neck
Auricular lymph node
Cervical lymph node
Facial lymph node
Jugular lymph node
Mandibular lymph node
Occipital lymph node
Parotid lymph node
Preauricular lymph node
Prelaryngeal lymph node
Pretracheal lymph node
Retropharyngeal lymph node
Scalene lymph node
Sublingual lymph node
Submandibular lymph node
Submaxillary lymph node
Submental lymph node
Supraclavicular lymph node

196.1 Intrathoracic lymph nodes
  Bronchial lymph node
  Bronchopulmonary lymph node
  Diaphragmatic lymph node
  Esophageal lymph node
  Hilar lymph node, NOS
  Innominate lymph node
  Intercostal lymph node
  Mediastinal lymph node
  Parasternal lymph node
  Pulmonary hilar lymph node
  Pulmonary lymph node, NOS
  Thoracic lymph node
  Tracheal lymph node
  Tracheobronchial lymph node

196.2 Intra-abdominal lymph nodes
  Abdominal lymph node
  Aortic lymph node
  Celiac lymph node
  Colic lymph node
  Common duct lymph node
  Gastric lymph node
  Hepatic lymph node
  Ileocolic lymph node
  Inferior mesenteric lymph node
  Intestinal lymph node
  Lumbar lymph node
  Mesenteric lymph node, NOS
  Midcolic lymph node
  Pancreatic lymph node
  Para-aortic lymph node
  Periaortic lymph node
  Peripancreatic lymph node
  Porta-hepatis lymph node
  Portal lymph node
  Pyloric lymph node
  Retroperitoneal lymph node
  Splenic lymph node, NOS
  Splenic hilar lymph node
  Superior mesenteric lymph node

196.3 Lymph nodes of axilla or arm
  Axillary lymph node
  Brachial lymph node
  Cubital lymph node
  Epitrochlear lymph node
  Infraclavicular lymph node
  Lymph node of upper limb
  Pectoral lymph node
  Subclavicular lymph node
  Subscapular lymph node

196.5 Lymph nodes of inguinal region or leg
  Femoral lymph node
  Inguinal lymph node
  Lymph node of Cloquet
  Lymph node of groin
  Lymph node of lower limb
  Lymph node of Rosenmüller
  Popliteal lymph node
  Subinguinal lymph node
  Tibial lymph node

196.6 Pelvic lymph nodes
  Hypogastric lymph node
  Iliac lymph node
  Inferior epigastric lymph node
  Intrapelvic lymph node
  Obturator lymph node
  Paracervical lymph node
  Parametrial lymph node
  Presymphysial lymph node
  Sacral lymph node

196.8 Lymph nodes of multiple regions

196.9 Lymph node, NOS

199 UNKNOWN PRIMARY SITE

199.9 Unknown primary site

5th DIGIT BEHAVIOR CODE FOR NEOPLASMS

/0 .... Benign

/1 .... Uncertain whether benign or malignant
Borderline malignancy

/2 .... Carcinoma-in-situ
Intraepithelial
Non-infiltrating
Non-invasive

/3 .... Malignant, primary site

/6 .... Malignant, metastatic site
Secondary site

/9 .... Malignant, uncertain whether primary or metastatic site

CODE FOR HISTOLOGIC GRADING AND DIFFERENTIATION

1 .... Grade I .... Well differentiated
Differentiated

2 .... Grade II .... Moderately differentiated
Moderately well differentiated

3 .... Grade III .... Poorly differentiated

4 .... Grade IV .... Undifferentiated
Anaplastic

9 .... Grade or differentiation not determined, not stated or
not applicable

MORPHOLOGY OF NEOPLASMS

NUMERICAL LIST

800 NEOPLASMS, NOS

8000/0 Neoplasm, benign
Tumor, benign
Unclassified tumor, benign

8000/1 Neoplasm, uncertain whether benign or malignant
Neoplasm, NOS
Tumor, NOS
Unclassified tumor, uncertain whether benign or malignant

8000/3 Neoplasm, malignant
Tumor, malignant, NOS
Malignancy
Cancer
Unclassified tumor, malignant

8000/6 Neoplasm, metastatic
Neoplasm, secondary
Tumor, metastatic
Tumor, secondary
Tumor embolus

8000/9 Neoplasm, malignant, uncertain whether primary or metastatic
Unclassified tumor, malignant, uncertain whether primary or metastatic

8001/0 Tumor cells, benign

8001/1 Tumor cells, uncertain whether benign or malignant
Tumor cells, NOS

8001/3 Tumor cells, malignant

8002/3 Malignant tumor, small cell type

8003/3 Malignant tumor, giant cell type

8004/3 Malignant tumor, fusiform cell type
Malignant tumor, spindle cell type

801-804 EPITHELIAL NEOPLASMS, NOS

8010/0 Epithelial tumor, benign

8010/2 Carcinoma-in-situ, NOS
Intraepithelial carcinoma, NOS

8010/3 Carcinoma, NOS
Epithelial tumor, malignant

8010/6 Carcinoma, metastatic, NOS
Secondary carcinoma

8010/9 Carcinomatosis

8011/0 Epithelioma, benign

8011/3 Epithelioma, malignant
Epithelioma, NOS

8012/3 Large cell carcinoma, NOS

8020/3 Carcinoma, undifferentiated type, NOS

8021/3 Carcinoma, anaplastic type, NOS

8022/3 Pleomorphic carcinoma

8030/3 Giant cell and spindle cell carcinoma

8031/3 Giant cell carcinoma

8032/3 Spindle cell carcinoma

8033/3 Pseudosarcomatous carcinoma

8034/3 Polygonal cell carcinoma

8035/3 Spheroidal cell carcinoma

8040/1 Tumorlet

8041/3 Small cell carcinoma, NOS
Reserve cell carcinoma
Round cell carcinoma

8042/3 Oat cell carcinoma (T-162._)

8043/3 Small cell carcinoma, fusiform cell type

805-808 PAPILLARY AND SQUAMOUS CELL NEOPLASMS

8050/0 Papilloma, NOS *(except Papilloma of urinary bladder M-8120/1)*

8050/2 Papillary carcinoma-in-situ

8050/3 Papillary carcinoma, NOS

8051/0 Verrucous papilloma

8051/3 Verrucous carcinoma, NOS
    Verrucous squamous cell carcinoma
    Verrucous epidermoid carcinoma

8052/0 Squamous cell papilloma
    Squamous papilloma
    Dyskeratotic papilloma
    Hyperkeratotic papilloma
    Keratotic papilloma
    Parakeratotic papilloma

8052/3 Papillary squamous cell carcinoma
    Papillary epidermoid carcinoma

8053/0 Inverted papilloma

8060/0 Papillomatosis, NOS

8070/2 Squamous cell carcinoma-in-situ, NOS
    Epidermoid carcinoma-in-situ, NOS
    Intraepidermal carcinoma, NOS
    Intraepithelial squamous cell carcinoma

8070/3 Squamous cell carcinoma, NOS
    Epidermoid carcinoma, NOS
    Spinous cell carcinoma
    Squamous carcinoma
    Squamous cell epithelioma

8070/6 Squamous cell carcinoma, metastatic, NOS

8071/3 Squamous cell carcinoma, keratinizing type, NOS
    Squamous cell carcinoma, large cell, keratinizing type
    Epidermoid carcinoma, keratinizing type

8072/3 Squamous cell carcinoma, large cell, non-keratinizing type
    Squamous cell carcinoma, non-keratinizing type, NOS
    Epidermoid carcinoma, large cell, non-keratinizing type

8073/3 Squamous cell carcinoma, small cell, non-keratinizing type
    Epidermoid carcinoma, small cell, non-keratinizing type

8074/3 Squamous cell carcinoma, spindle cell type
    Epidermoid carcinoma, spindle cell type

8075/3 Adenoid squamous cell carcinoma
    Pseudoglandular squamous cell carcinoma

8076/2 Squamous cell carcinoma-in-situ with questionable stromal invasion (T-180._)
    Epidermoid carcinoma-in-situ with questionable stromal invasion (T-180._)

8076/3 Squamous cell carcinoma, micro-invasive (T-180._)

8080/2 Queyrat's erythroplasia (T-187._)

8081/2 Bowen's disease (T-173._)
    Intraepidermal squamous cell carcinoma, Bowen's type (T-173._)

8082/3 Lymphoepithelial carcinoma
    Lymphoepithelioma

809-811 BASAL CELL NEOPLASMS

8090/1 Basal cell tumor (T-173._)

8090/3 Basal cell carcinoma, NOS (T-173._)
    Pigmented basal cell carcinoma (T-173._)
    Basal cell epithelioma (T-173._)
    Rodent ulcer (T-173._)

8091/3 Multicentric basal cell carcinoma (T-173._)

8092/3 Basal cell carcinoma, morphea type (T-173._)

8093/3 Basal cell carcinoma, fibroepithelial type (T-173._)

8094/3 Basosquamous carcinoma (T-173._)
    Mixed basal-squamous cell carcinoma
    (T-173._)

8095/3 Metatypical carcinoma (T-173._)

8096/0 Intraepidermal epithelioma of Jadassohn
    (T-173._)

8100/0 Trichoepithelioma (T-173._)
    Brooke's tumor (T-173._)
    Epithelioma adenoides cysticum (T-173._)

8101/0 Trichofolliculoma (T-173._)

8102/0 Tricholemmoma (T-173._)

8110/0 Pilomatrixoma (T-173._)
    Calcifying epithelioma of Malherbe
    (T-173._)

812-813 TRANSITIONAL CELL PAPILLOMAS AND CARCINOMAS

8120/0 Transitional cell papilloma, NOS
    Transitional papilloma

8120/1 Urothelial papilloma
    Papilloma of urinary bladder (T-188._)

8120/2 Transitional cell carcinoma-in-situ

8120/3 Transitional cell carcinoma, NOS
    Transitional carcinoma
    Urothelial carcinoma

8121/0 Schneiderian papilloma

8121/1 Transitional cell papilloma, inverted type

8121/3 Schneiderian carcinoma

8122/3 Transitional cell carcinoma, spindle cell type

8123/3 Basaloid carcinoma

8124/3 Cloacogenic carcinoma

8130/3 Papillary transitional cell carcinoma

814-838 ADENOMAS AND ADENOCARCINOMAS

8140/0 Adenoma, NOS

8140/1 Bronchial adenoma, NOS (T-162._)

8140/2 Adenocarcinoma-in-situ

8140/3 Adenocarcinoma, NOS

8140/6 Adenocarcinoma, metastatic, NOS

8141/3 Scirrhous adenocarcinoma
    Scirrhous carcinoma
    Carcinoma with productive fibrosis

8142/3 Linitis plastica (T-151._)

8143/3 Superficial spreading adenocarcinoma

8144/3 Adenocarcinoma, intestinal type (T-151._)
    Carcinoma, intestinal type (T-151._)

8145/3 Carcinoma, diffuse type (T-151._)
    Adenocarcinoma, diffuse type (T-151._)

8146/0 Monomorphic adenoma

8147/0 Basal cell adenoma

8150/0 Islet cell adenoma (T-157._)
    Islet cell tumor (T-157._)
    Nesidioblastoma (T-157._)

8150/3 Islet cell carcinoma (T-157._)
    Islet cell adenocarcinoma (T-157._)

8151/0 Insulinoma, NOS (T-157._)
    Beta-cell adenoma (T-157._)

8151/3 Insulinoma, malignant (T-157._)
    Beta-cell tumor, malignant (T-157._)

8152/0 Glucagonoma, NOS (T-157._)
    Alpha-cell adenoma (T-157._)

8152/3 Glucagonoma, malignant (T-157._)
    Alpha-cell tumor, malignant (T-157._)

8153/1 Gastrinoma, NOS
    G cell tumor, NOS

8153/3 Gastrinoma, malignant
    G cell tumor, malignant

8154/3 Mixed islet cell and exocrine adenocarcinoma (T-157._)

8160/0 Bile duct adenoma (T-155._)
    Cholangioma (T-155._)

8160/3 Cholangiocarcinoma (T-155._)
    Bile duct carcinoma (T-155._)
    Bile duct adenocarcinoma (T-155._)

8161/0 Bile duct cystadenoma (T-155._)

8161/3 Bile duct cystadenocarcinoma (T-155._)

8170/0 Liver cell adenoma (T-155.0)
    Hepatocellular adenoma (T-155.0)
    Hepatoma, benign (T-155.0)

8170/3 Hepatocellular carcinoma, NOS (T-155.0)
    Liver cell carcinoma (T-155.0)
    Hepatocarcinoma (T-155.0)
    Hepatoma, malignant (T-155.0)
    Hepatoma, NOS (T-155.0)

8180/0 Hepatocholangioma, benign (T-155.0)

8180/3 Combined hepatocellular carcinoma and cholangiocarcinoma (T-155.0)
    Mixed hepatocellular and bile duct carcinoma (T-155.0)
    Hepatocholangiocarcinoma (T-155.0)

8190/0 Trabecular adenoma

8190/3 Trabecular adenocarcinoma
    Trabecular carcinoma

8191/0 Embryonal adenoma

8200/0 Eccrine dermal cylindroma (T-173._)
    Turban tumor (T-173.4)
    Cylindroma of skin (T-173._)

8200/3 Adenoid cystic carcinoma
    Adenocystic carcinoma
    Cylindroma, NOS (except Cylindroma of skin M-8200/0)
    Bronchial adenoma, cylindroid type (T-162._)
    Adenocarcinoma, cylindroid type

8201/3 Cribriform carcinoma

8210/0 Adenomatous polyp, NOS
    Polypoid adenoma

8210/3 Adenocarcinoma in adenomatous polyp
    Adenocarcinoma in tubular adenoma
    Carcinoma in adenomatous polyp
    Adenocarcinoma in polypoid adenoma

8211/0 Tubular adenoma, NOS

8211/3 Tubular adenocarcinoma
    Tubular carcinoma

8220/0 Adenomatous polyposis coli (T-153._)
    Adenomatosis, NOS (T-153._)
    Familial polyposis coli (T-153._)

8220/3 Adenocarcinoma in adenomatous polyposis coli (T-153._)

8221/0 Multiple adenomatous polyps
    Multiple polyposis

8230/3 Solid carcinoma, NOS

8231/3 Carcinoma simplex

8240/1 Carcinoid tumor, NOS
    Carcinoid, NOS

8240/3 Carcinoid tumor, malignant
    Carcinoid, malignant
    Bronchial adenoma, carcinoid type (T-162._)

8241/1 Carcinoid tumor, argentaffin, NOS
    Argentaffinoma, NOS

8241/3 Carcinoid tumor, argentaffin, malignant
    Argentaffinoma, malignant

8242/1 Carcinoid tumor, non-argentaffin, NOS

8242/3 Carcinoid tumor, non-argentaffin, malignant

8243/3 Mucocarcinoid tumor, malignant
    Goblet cell carcinoid

8244/3 Composite carcinoid

8250/1 Pulmonary adenomatosis (T-162._)

8250/3 Bronchiolo-alveolar adenocarcinoma (T-162._)
    Alveolar cell carcinoma (T-162._)
    Bronchiolo-alveolar carcinoma (T-162._)
    Bronchiolar adenocarcinoma (T-162._)
    Bronchiolar carcinoma (T-162._)
    Terminal bronchiolar carcinoma (T-162._)

8251/0 Alveolar adenoma

8251/3 Alveolar adenocarcinoma
    Alveolar carcinoma

8260/0 Papillary adenoma, NOS

8260/3 Papillary adenocarcinoma, NOS

8261/1 Villous adenoma, NOS
    Villous papilloma

8261/3 Adenocarcinoma in villous adenoma

8262/3 Villous adenocarcinoma

8263/0 Tubulovillous adenoma
    Villoglandular adenoma
    Papillotubular adenoma

8270/0 Chromophobe adenoma (T-194.3)

8270/3 Chromophobe carcinoma (T-194.3)
    Chromophobe adenocarcinoma (T-194.3)

8280/0 Acidophil adenoma (T-194.3)
    Eosinophil adenoma (T-194.3)

8280/3 Acidophil carcinoma (T-194.3)
    Acidophil adenocarcinoma (T-194.3)
    Eosinophil carcinoma (T-194.3)
    Eosinophil adenocarcinoma (T-194.3)

8281/0 Mixed acidophil-basophil adenoma (T-194.3)

8281/3 Mixed acidophil-basophil carcinoma (T-194.3)

8290/0 Oxyphilic adenoma
    Oncocytic adenoma
    Oncocytoma
    Hürthle cell adenoma (T-193.9)
    Hürthle cell tumor (T-193.9)

8290/3 Oxyphilic adenocarcinoma
    Oncocytic carcinoma
    Oncocytic adenocarcinoma
    Hürthle cell carcinoma (T-193.9)
    Hürthle cell adenocarcinoma (T-193.9)

8300/0 Basophil adenoma (T-194.3)
    Mucoid cell adenoma (T-194.3)

8300/3 Basophil carcinoma (T-194.3)
    Basophil adenocarcinoma (T-194.3)
    Mucoid cell adenocarcinoma (T-194.3)

8310/0 Clear cell adenoma

8310/3 Clear cell adenocarcinoma, NOS
    Clear cell adenocarcinoma, mesonephroid
        type
    Clear cell carcinoma

8311/1 Hypernephroid tumor

8312/3 Renal cell carcinoma (T-189.0)
    Renal cell adenocarcinoma (T-189.0)
    Grawitz tumor (T-189.0)
    Hypernephroma (T-189.0)

8313/0 Clear cell adenofibroma
    Clear cell cystadenofibroma

8320/3 Granular cell carcinoma
    Granular cell adenocarcinoma

8321/0 Chief cell adenoma (T-194.1)

8322/0 Water-clear cell adenoma (T-194.1)

8322/3 Water-clear cell adenocarcinoma (T-194.1)
    Water-clear cell carcinoma (T-194.1)

8323/0 Mixed cell adenoma

8323/3 Mixed cell adenocarcinoma

8324/0 Lipoadenoma

8330/0 Follicular adenoma (T-193.9)

8330/3 Follicular adenocarcinoma, NOS (T-193.9)
    Follicular carcinoma, NOS (T-193.9)

8331/3 Follicular adenocarcinoma, well differentiated type (T-193.9)
Follicular carcinoma, well differentiated type (T-193.9)
Follicular adenocarcinoma, pure follicle type (T-193.9)
Follicular carcinoma, pure follicle type (T-193.9)

8332/3 Follicular adenocarcinoma, trabecular type (T-193.9)
Follicular carcinoma, trabecular type (T-193.9)
Follicular adenocarcinoma, moderately differentiated type (T-193.9)
Follicular carcinoma, moderately differentiated type (T-193.9)
Wuchernde Struma Langhans (T-193.9)

8333/0 Microfollicular adenoma (T-193.9)
Fetal adenoma (T-193.9)

8334/0 Macrofollicular adenoma (T-193.9)
Colloid adenoma (T-193.9)

8340/3 Papillary and follicular adenocarcinoma (T-193.9)
Papillary and follicular carcinoma (T-193.9)
Mixed papillary and follicular carcinoma (T-193.9)

8350/3 Nonencapsulated sclerosing carcinoma (T-193.9)
Nonencapsulated sclerosing adenocarcinoma (T-193.9)
Nonencapsulated sclerosing tumor (T-193.9)

8360/1 Multiple endocrine adenomas
Endocrine adenomatosis

8361/1 Juxtaglomerular tumor (T-189.0)
Reninoma (T-189.0)

8370/0 Adrenal cortical adenoma, NOS (T-194.0)
Adrenal cortical tumor, benign (T-194.0)
Adrenal cortical tumor, NOS (T-194.0)

8370/3 Adrenal cortical carcinoma (T-194.0)
Adrenal cortical adenocarcinoma (T-194.0)
Adrenal cortical tumor, malignant (T-194.0)

8371/0 Adrenal cortical adenoma, compact cell type (T-194.0)

8372/0 Adrenal cortical adenoma, heavily pigmented variant (T-194.0)
Black adenoma (T-194.0)

8373/0 Adrenal cortical adenoma, clear cell type (T-194.0)

8374/0 Adrenal cortical adenoma, glomerulosa cell type (T-194.0)

8375/0 Adrenal cortical adenoma, mixed cell type (T-194.0)

8380/0 Endometrioid adenoma, NOS
Endometrioid cystadenoma, NOS

8380/1 Endometrioid adenoma, borderline malignancy
Endometrioid cystadenoma, borderline malignancy

8380/3 Endometrioid carcinoma
Endometrioid adenocarcinoma
Endometrioid cystadenocarcinoma

8381/0 Endometrioid adenofibroma, NOS (T-183.0)
Endometrioid cystadenofibroma, NOS (T-183.0)

8381/1 Endometrioid adenofibroma, borderline malignancy (T-183.0)
Endometrioid cystadenofibroma, borderline malignancy (T-183.0)

8381/3 Endometrioid adenofibroma, malignant (T-183.0)
Endometrioid cystadenofibroma, malignant (T-183.0)

839-842 ADNEXAL AND SKIN APPENDAGE NEOPLASMS

8390/0 Skin appendage adenoma (T-173._)
Skin appendage tumor (T-173._)
Adnexal tumor (T-173._)

8390/3 Skin appendage carcinoma (T-173._)
Adnexal carcinoma (T-173._)

8400/0 **Sweat gland adenoma (T-173.__)**
    Sweat gland tumor, benign (T-173.__)
    Hidradenoma, NOS (T-173.__)
    Syringadenoma, NOS (T-173.__)
    Nodular hidradenoma (T-173.__)

8400/1 **Sweat gland tumor, NOS (T-173.__)**

8400/3 **Sweat gland adenocarcinoma (T-173.__)**
    Sweat gland carcinoma (T-173.__)
    Sweat gland tumor, malignant (T-173.__)

8401/0 **Apocrine adenoma**

8401/3 **Apocrine adenocarcinoma**

8402/0 **Eccrine acrospiroma (T-173.__)**
    Eccrine poroma (T-173.__)
    Clear cell hidradenoma (T-173.__)

8403/0 **Eccrine spiradenoma (T-173.__)**
    Spiradenoma, NOS (T-173.__)

8404/0 **Hidrocystoma (T-173.__)**

8405/0 **Papillary hidradenoma (T-173.__)**

8406/0 **Papillary syringadenoma (T-173.__)**
    Papillary syringocystadenoma (T-173.__)

8407/0 **Syringoma, NOS (T-173.__)**

8410/0 **Sebaceous adenoma (T-173.__)**

8410/3 **Sebaceous adenocarcinoma (T-173.__)**
    Sebaceous carcinoma (T-173.__)

8420/0 **Ceruminous adenoma (T-173.2)**

8420/3 **Ceruminous adenocarcinoma (T-173.2)**
    Ceruminous carcinoma (T-173.2)

843 MUCOEPIDERMOID NEOPLASMS

8430/1 **Mucoepidermoid tumor**

8430/3 **Mucoepidermoid carcinoma**

844-849 CYSTIC, MUCINOUS AND SEROUS NEOPLASMS

8440/0 **Cystadenoma, NOS**
    Cystoma, NOS

8440/3 **Cystadenocarcinoma, NOS**

8441/0 **Serous cystadenoma, NOS (T-183.0)**
    Serous cystoma (T-183.0)

8441/1 **Serous cystadenoma, borderline malignancy (T-183.0)**

8441/3 **Serous cystadenocarcinoma, NOS (T-183.0)**
    Serous adenocarcinoma, NOS

8450/0 **Papillary cystadenoma, NOS (T-183.0)**

8450/1 **Papillary cystadenoma, borderline malignancy (T-183.0)**

8450/3 **Papillary cystadenocarcinoma, NOS (T-183.0)**
    Papillocystic adenocarcinoma

8460/0 **Papillary serous cystadenoma, NOS (T-183.0)**

8460/1 **Papillary serous cystadenoma, borderline malignancy (T-183.0)**

8460/3 **Papillary serous cystadenocarcinoma (T-183.0)**
    Papillary serous adenocarcinoma (T-183.0)

8461/0 **Serous surface papilloma, NOS (T-183.0)**

8461/1 **Serous surface papilloma, borderline malignancy (T-183.0)**

8461/3 **Serous surface papillary carcinoma (T-183.0)**

8470/0 **Mucinous cystadenoma, NOS (T-183.0)**
    Mucinous cystoma (T-183.0)
    Pseudomucinous cystadenoma, NOS (T-183.0)

8470/1 **Mucinous cystadenoma, borderline malignancy (T-183.0)**
    Pseudomucinous cystadenoma, borderline malignancy (T-183.0)

8470/3 **Mucinous cystadenocarcinoma, NOS (T-183.0)**
   Pseudomucinous adenocarcinoma (T-183.0)
   Pseudomucinous cystadenocarcinoma, NOS
      (T-183.0)

8471/0 **Papillary mucinous cystadenoma, NOS**
      (T-183.0)
   Papillary pseudomucinous cystadenoma,
      NOS (T-183.0)

8471/1 **Papillary mucinous cystadenoma, borderline**
      malignancy (T-183.0)
   Papillary pseudomucinous cystadenoma,
      borderline malignancy (T-183.0)

8471/3 **Papillary mucinous cystadenocarcinoma**
      (T-183.0)
   Papillary pseudomucinous
      cystadenocarcinoma (T-183.0)

8480/0 **Mucinous adenoma**

8480/3 **Mucinous adenocarcinoma**
   Mucinous carcinoma
   Colloid adenocarcinoma
   Colloid carcinoma
   Gelatinous adenocarcinoma
   Gelatinous carcinoma
   Mucoid adenocarcinoma
   Mucoid carcinoma
   Mucous adenocarcinoma
   Mucous carcinoma

8480/6 **Pseudomyxoma peritonei (T-158.9)**

8481/3 **Mucin-producing adenocarcinoma**
   Mucin-producing carcinoma
   Mucin-secreting adenocarcinoma
   Mucin-secreting carcinoma

8490/3 **Signet ring cell carcinoma**
   Signet ring cell adenocarcinoma

8490/6 **Metastatic signet ring cell carcinoma**
   Krukenberg tumor (T-183.0)

850-854 DUCTAL, LOBULAR AND MEDULLARY NEOPLASMS

8500/2 **Intraductal carcinoma, non-infiltrating, NOS**
   Intraductal adenocarcinoma, non-
      infiltrating, NOS
   Intraduct carcinoma-in-situ
   Intraductal carcinoma, NOS

8500/3 **Infiltrating duct carcinoma (T-174._)**
   Infiltrating duct adenocarcinoma (T-174._)
   Duct adenocarcinoma, NOS
   Duct carcinoma, NOS
   Duct cell carcinoma
   Ductal carcinoma

8501/2 **Comedocarcinoma, non-infiltrating (T-174._)**

8501/3 **Comedocarcinoma, NOS (T-174._)**

8502/3 **Juvenile carcinoma of the breast (T-174._)**
   Secretory carcinoma of the breast
      (T-174._)

8503/0 **Intraductal papilloma**
   Duct adenoma, NOS
   Ductal papilloma

8503/2 **Non-infiltrating intraductal papillary**
      adenocarcinoma
   Non-infiltrating intraductal papillary
      carcinoma

8504/0 **Intracystic papillary adenoma**
   Intracystic papilloma

8504/2 **Non-infiltrating intracystic carcinoma**

8505/0 **Intraductal papillomatosis, NOS**
   Diffuse intraductal papillomatosis

8506/0 **Subareolar duct papillomatosis (T-174.0)**
   Erosive adenomatosis of the nipple
      (T-174.0)
   Adenoma of the nipple (T-174.0)

8510/3 **Medullary carcinoma, NOS**
   Medullary adenocarcinoma
   Parafollicular cell carcinoma (T-193.9)
   C cell carcinoma (T-193.9)

8511/3 Medullary carcinoma with amyloid stroma (T-193.9)
Solid carcinoma with amyloid stroma (T-193.9)

8512/3 Medullary carcinoma with lymphoid stroma (T-174.__)

8520/2 Lobular carcinoma-in-situ (T-174.__)
Lobular carcinoma, non-infiltrating (T-174.__)

8520/3 Lobular carcinoma, NOS (T-174.__)
Lobular adenocarcinoma (T-174.__)
Infiltrating lobular carcinoma (T-174.__)

8521/3 Infiltrating ductular carcinoma

8530/3 Inflammatory carcinoma (T-174.__)
Inflammatory adenocarcinoma (T-174.__)

8540/3 Paget's disease, mammary (T-174.__)
Paget's disease of breast (T-174.__)

8541/3 Paget's disease and infiltrating duct carcinoma of breast (T-174.__)

8542/3 Paget's disease, extramammary *(except Paget's disease of bone)*

855 ACINAR CELL NEOPLASMS

8550/0 Acinar cell adenoma
Acinar adenoma
Acinic cell adenoma

8550/1 Acinar cell tumor
Acinic cell tumor

8550/3 Acinar cell carcinoma
Acinic cell adenocarcinoma
Acinar adenocarcinoma
Acinar carcinoma

856-858 COMPLEX EPITHELIAL NEOPLASMS

8560/3 Adenosquamous carcinoma
Mixed adenocarcinoma and squamous cell carcinoma
Mixed adenocarcinoma and epidermoid carcinoma

8561/0 Adenolymphoma (T-142.__)
Papillary cystadenoma lymphomatosum (T-142.__)
Warthin's tumor (T-142.__)

8570/3 Adenocarcinoma with squamous metaplasia
Adenoacanthoma

8571/3 Adenocarcinoma with cartilaginous and osseous metaplasia
Adenocarcinoma with cartilaginous metaplasia
Adenocarcinoma with osseous metaplasia

8572/3 Adenocarcinoma with spindle cell metaplasia

8573/3 Adenocarcinoma with apocrine metaplasia
Carcinoma with apocrine metaplasia

8580/0 Thymoma, benign (T-164.0)
Thymoma, NOS (T-164.0)

8580/3 Thymoma, malignant (T-164.0)
Thymic carcinoma (T-164.0)

859-867 SPECIALIZED GONADAL NEOPLASMS

8590/1 Sex cord-stromal tumor
Gonadal stromal tumor
Testicular stromal tumor (T-186.__)
Ovarian stromal tumor (T-183.0)
Sex cord tumor

8600/0 Thecoma, NOS (T-183.0)
Theca cell tumor (T-183.0)

8600/3 Theca cell carcinoma (T-183.0)
Thecoma, malignant (T-183.0)

8610/0 Luteoma, NOS (T-183.0)
Luteinoma (T-183.0)

8620/1 Granulosa cell tumor, NOS (T-183.0)

8620/3 Granulosa cell tumor, malignant (T-183.0)
Granulosa cell carcinoma (T-183.0)

8621/1 Granulosa cell-theca cell tumor (T-183.0)
Theca cell-granulosa cell tumor (T-183.0)

8630/0 Androblastoma, benign
Arrhenoblastoma, benign

8630/1 **Androblastoma, NOS**
    Arrhenoblastoma, NOS

8630/3 **Androblastoma, malignant**
    Arrhenoblastoma, malignant

8631/0 **Sertoli-Leydig cell tumor**

8632/1 **Gynandroblastoma (T-183.0)**

8640/0 **Tubular androblastoma, NOS**
    Pick's tubular adenoma
    Sertoli cell adenoma
    Sertoli cell tumor, NOS
    Testicular adenoma

8640/3 **Sertoli cell carcinoma (T-186.__)**

8641/0 **Tubular androblastoma with lipid storage (T-183.0)**
    Sertoli cell tumor with lipid storage

8650/0 **Leydig cell tumor, benign (T-186.__)**
    Interstitial cell tumor, benign

8650/1 **Leydig cell tumor, NOS (T-186.__)**
    Interstitial cell tumor, NOS

8650/3 **Leydig cell tumor, malignant (T-186.__)**
    Interstitial cell tumor, malignant

8660/0 **Hilar cell tumor (T-183.0)**

8670/0 **Lipid cell tumor of ovary (T-183.0)**
    Lipoid cell tumor of ovary (T-183.0)
    Masculinovoblastoma (T-183.0)

8671/0 **Adrenal rest tumor**

868-871 PARAGANGLIOMAS AND GLOMUS TUMORS

8680/1 **Paraganglioma, NOS**

8680/3 **Paraganglioma, malignant**

8681/1 **Sympathetic paraganglioma**

8682/1 **Parasympathetic paraganglioma**

8690/1 **Glomus jugulare tumor (T-194.6)**
    Jugular paraganglioma (T-194.6)

8691/1 **Aortic body tumor (T-194.6)**
    Aortic body paraganglioma (T-194.6)

8692/1 **Carotid body tumor (T-194.5)**
    Carotid body paraganglioma (T-194.5)

8693/1 **Extra-adrenal paraganglioma, NOS**
    Nonchromaffin paraganglioma, NOS
    Chemodectoma

8693/3 **Extra-adrenal paraganglioma, malignant**
    Nonchromaffin paraganglioma, malignant

8700/0 **Pheochromocytoma, NOS (T-194.0)**
    Chromaffin paraganglioma
    Chromaffin tumor
    Chromaffinoma

8700/3 **Pheochromocytoma, malignant (T-194.0)**
    Pheochromoblastoma (T-194.0)

8710/3 **Glomangiosarcoma**
    Glomoid sarcoma

8711/0 **Glomus tumor**

8712/0 **Glomangioma**

872-879 NEVI AND MELANOMAS

8720/0 **Pigmented nevus, NOS (T-173.__)**
    Nevus, NOS (T-173.__)
    Hairy nevus (T-173.__)

8720/3 **Malignant melanoma, NOS**
    Melanoma, NOS
    Melanocarcinoma
    Nevocarcinoma
    Melanosarcoma, NOS

8721/3 **Nodular melanoma**

8722/0 **Balloon cell nevus (T-173.__)**

8722/3 **Balloon cell melanoma**

8723/0 **Halo nevus (T-173.__)**

8724/0 **Fibrous papule of the nose (T-173.3)**
    Involuting nevus (T-173.__)

8725/0 Neuronevus (T-173.__)

8726/0 Magnocellular nevus (T-190.0)
    Melanocytoma of the eyeball (T-190.0)

8730/0 Non-pigmented nevus (T-173.__)
    Achromic nevus (T-173.__)

8730/3 Amelanotic melanoma

8740/0 Junctional nevus (T-173.__)
    Junction nevus (T-173.__)
    Intraepidermal nevus (T-173.__)

8740/3 Malignant melanoma in junctional nevus
    (T-173.__)

8741/2 Precancerous melanosis, NOS (T-173.__)

8741/3 Malignant melanoma in precancerous
    melanosis (T-173.__)

8742/2 Hutchinson's melanotic freckle (T-173.__)
    Lentigo maligna (T-173.__)

8742/3 Malignant melanoma in Hutchinson's
    melanotic freckle (T-173.__)
    Lentigo maligna melanoma (T-173.__)

8743/3 Superficial spreading melanoma

8750/0 Intradermal nevus (T-173.__)
    Dermal nevus (T-173.__)

8760/0 Compound nevus (T-173.__)
    Dermal and epidermal nevus (T-173.__)

8761/1 Giant pigmented nevus (T-173.__)

8761/3 Malignant melanoma in giant pigmented
    nevus (T-173.__)

8770/0 Epithelioid and spindle cell nevus (T-173.__)
    Epithelioid cell nevus (T-173.__)
    Spindle cell nevus (T-173.__)
    Juvenile nevus (T-173.__)
    Juvenile melanoma (T-173.__)

8771/3 Epithelioid cell melanoma
    Epithelioid cell melanosarcoma

8772/3 Spindle cell melanoma, NOS

8773/3 Spindle cell melanoma, type A (T-190.0)

8774/3 Spindle cell melanoma, type B (T-190.0)

8775/3 Mixed epithelioid and spindle cell melanoma

8780/0 Blue nevus, NOS (T-173.__)
    Jadassohn's blue nevus (T-173.__)

8780/3 Blue nevus, malignant (T-173.__)

8790/0 Cellular blue nevus (T-173.__)
    Giant blue nevus (T-173.__)

880 SOFT TISSUE TUMORS AND SARCOMAS, NOS

8800/0 Soft tissue tumor, benign

8800/3 Sarcoma, NOS
    Soft tissue tumor, malignant
    Mesenchymal tumor, malignant

8800/9 Sarcomatosis, NOS

8801/3 Spindle cell sarcoma

8802/3 Giant cell sarcoma *(except of Bone M-9250/3)*
    Pleomorphic cell sarcoma

8803/3 Small cell sarcoma
    Round cell sarcoma

8804/3 Epithelioid cell sarcoma

881-883 FIBROMATOUS NEOPLASMS

8810/0 Fibroma, NOS
    Fibroma durum

8810/3 Fibrosarcoma, NOS

8811/0 Fibromyxoma
    Myxoid fibroma
    Myxofibroma, NOS

8811/3 Fibromyxosarcoma

8812/0 Periosteal fibroma (T-170.__)

8812/3 **Periosteal fibrosarcoma (T-170._)**
  Periosteal sarcoma, NOS **(T-170._)**

8813/0 **Fascial fibroma**

8813/3 **Fascial fibrosarcoma**

8814/3 **Infantile fibrosarcoma**
  Congenital fibrosarcoma

8820/0 **Elastofibroma**

8821/1 **Aggressive fibromatosis**
  Extra-abdominal desmoid
  Desmoid, NOS
  Invasive fibroma

8822/1 **Abdominal fibromatosis**
  Abdominal desmoid

8823/1 **Desmoplastic fibroma**

8830/0 **Fibrous histiocytoma, NOS**

8830/1 **Atypical fibrous histiocytoma**

8830/3 **Fibrous histiocytoma, malignant**

8831/0 **Fibroxanthoma, NOS**
  Xanthofibroma

8831/1 **Atypical fibroxanthoma**

8831/3 **Fibroxanthoma, malignant**
  Fibroxanthosarcoma

8832/0 **Dermatofibroma, NOS (T-173._)**
  Sclerosing hemangioma **(T-173._)**
  Histiocytoma, NOS **(T-173._)**
  Subepidermal nodular fibrosis **(T-173._)**
  Dermatofibroma lenticulare **(T-173._)**

8832/1 **Dermatofibroma protuberans (T-173._)**

8832/3 **Dermatofibrosarcoma, NOS (T-173._)**
  Dermatofibrosarcoma protuberans **(T-173._)**

884 MYXOMATOUS NEOPLASMS

8840/0 **Myxoma, NOS**

8840/3 **Myxosarcoma**

885-888 LIPOMATOUS NEOPLASMS

8850/0 **Lipoma, NOS**

8850/3 **Liposarcoma, NOS**
  Fibroliposarcoma

8851/0 **Fibrolipoma**
  Fibroma molle
  Soft fibroma

8851/3 **Liposarcoma, well differentiated type**
  Liposarcoma, differentiated type

8852/0 **Fibromyxolipoma**
  Myxolipoma

8852/3 **Myxoid liposarcoma**
  Myxoliposarcoma
  Embryonal liposarcoma

8853/3 **Round cell liposarcoma**

8854/3 **Pleomorphic liposarcoma**

8855/3 **Mixed type liposarcoma**

8856/0 **Intramuscular lipoma**
  Infiltrating lipoma

8857/0 **Spindle cell lipoma**

8860/0 **Angiomyolipoma**

8860/3 **Angiomyoliposarcoma**

8861/0 **Angiolipoma, NOS**

8861/1 **Angiolipoma, infiltrating**

8870/0 **Myelolipoma**

8880/0 **Hibernoma**
    Fetal fat cell lipoma
    Brown fat tumor

8881/0 **Lipoblastomatosis**
    Fetal lipoma, NOS
    Fetal lipomatosis
    Lipoblastoma

889-892 MYOMATOUS NEOPLASMS

8890/0 **Leiomyoma, NOS**
    Fibroid uterus (T-179.9)
    Fibromyoma
    Leiomyofibroma
    Myofibroma

8890/1 **Intravascular leiomyomatosis**

8890/3 **Leiomyosarcoma, NOS**

8891/1 **Epithelioid leiomyoma**
    Leiomyoblastoma

8891/3 **Epithelioid leiomyosarcoma**

8892/1 **Cellular leiomyoma**

8893/0 **Bizarre leiomyoma**

8894/0 **Angiomyoma**
    Vascular leiomyoma
    Angioleiomyoma

8894/3 **Angiomyosarcoma**

8895/0 **Myoma**

8895/3 **Myosarcoma**

8900/0 **Rhabdomyoma, NOS**

8900/3 **Rhabdomyosarcoma, NOS**
    Rhabdosarcoma

8901/3 **Pleomorphic rhabdomyosarcoma**

8902/3 **Mixed type rhabdomyosarcoma**

8903/0 **Fetal rhabdomyoma**

8904/0 **Adult rhabdomyoma**
    Glycogenic rhabdomyoma

8910/3 **Embryonal rhabdomyosarcoma**
    Sarcoma botryoides
    Botryoid sarcoma

8920/3 **Alveolar rhabdomyosarcoma**

893-899 COMPLEX MIXED AND STROMAL NEOPLASMS

8930/3 **Endometrial stromal sarcoma (T-182.0)**
    Endometrial sarcoma, NOS (T-182.0)
    Stromal sarcoma, NOS

8931/1 **Endolymphatic stromal myosis (T-182.0)**
    Endometrial stromatosis (T-182.0)
    Stromal endometriosis (T-182.0)
    Stromal myosis, NOS (T-182.0)

8932/0 **Adenomyoma**

8940/0 **Pleomorphic adenoma**
    Mixed tumor, NOS
    Mixed tumor, salivary gland type, NOS
    Chondroid syringoma

8940/3 **Mixed tumor, malignant, NOS**
    Mixed tumor, salivary gland type,
      malignant
    Carcinoma in pleomorphic adenoma

8950/3 **Müllerian mixed tumor**

8951/3 **Mesodermal mixed tumor**

8960/1 **Mesoblastic nephroma**

8960/3 **Nephroblastoma, NOS (T-189.0)**
    Wilms's tumor (T-189.0)
    Adenosarcoma (T-189.0)

8961/3 **Epithelial nephroblastoma (T-189.0)**

8962/3 **Mesenchymal nephroblastoma (T-189.0)**

8970/3 **Hepatoblastoma (T-155.0)**
    Embryonal hepatoma (T-155.0)

8980/3 **Carcinosarcoma, NOS**

8981/3 **Carcinosarcoma, embryonal type**
Pneumoblastoma (T-162._)

8982/0 **Myoepithelioma**
Myoepithelial tumor

8990/0 **Mesenchymoma, benign**

8990/1 **Mesenchymoma, NOS**
Mixed mesenchymal tumor

8990/3 **Mesenchymoma, malignant**
Mixed mesenchymal sarcoma

8991/3 **Embryonal sarcoma**

900-903 FIBROEPITHELIAL NEOPLASMS

9000/0 **Brenner tumor, NOS (T-183.0)**

9000/1 **Brenner tumor, borderline malignancy (T-183.0)**
Brenner tumor, proliferating (T-183.0)

9000/3 **Brenner tumor, malignant (T-183.0)**

9010/0 **Fibroadenoma, NOS (T-174._)**

9011/0 **Intracanalicular fibroadenoma, NOS (T-174._)**

9012/0 **Pericanalicular fibroadenoma (T-174._)**

9013/0 **Adenofibroma, NOS (T-183.0)**
Cystadenofibroma, NOS (T-183.0)

9014/0 **Serous adenofibroma (T-183.0)**
Serous cystadenofibroma (T-183.0)

9015/0 **Mucinous adenofibroma (T-183.0)**
Mucinous cystadenofibroma (T-183.0)

9020/0 **Cellular intracanalicular fibroadenoma (T-174._)**
Fibroadenoma phyllodes (T-174._)
Giant fibroadenoma, NOS (T-174._)
Giant intracanalicular fibroadenoma (T-174._)
Cystosarcoma phyllodes, benign (T-174._)

9020/1 **Cystosarcoma phyllodes, NOS (T-174._)**

9020/3 **Cystosarcoma phyllodes, malignant (T-174._)**

9030/0 **Juvenile fibroadenoma (T-174._)**

904 SYNOVIAL NEOPLASMS

9040/0 **Synovioma, benign**

9040/3 **Synovial sarcoma, NOS**
Synovioma, NOS
Synovioma, malignant

9041/3 **Synovial sarcoma, spindle cell type**

9042/3 **Synovial sarcoma, epithelioid cell type**

9043/3 **Synovial sarcoma, biphasic type**

9044/3 **Clear cell sarcoma of tendons and aponeuroses (T-171._)**

905 MESOTHELIAL NEOPLASMS

9050/0 **Mesothelioma, benign**

9050/3 **Mesothelioma, malignant**
Mesothelioma, NOS
Mesothelial sarcoma

9051/0 **Fibrous mesothelioma, benign**

9051/3 **Fibrous mesothelioma, malignant**
Fibrous mesothelioma, NOS

9052/0 **Epithelioid mesothelioma, benign**

9052/3 **Epithelioid mesothelioma, malignant**
Epithelioid mesothelioma, NOS

9053/0 **Mesothelioma, biphasic type, benign**

9053/3 **Mesothelioma, biphasic type, malignant**
Mesothelioma, biphasic type, NOS

9054/0 **Adenomatoid tumor, NOS**

906-909 GERM CELL NEOPLASMS

9060/3 Dysgerminoma

9061/3 Seminoma, NOS (T-186._)

9062/3 Seminoma, anaplastic type (T-186._)

9063/3 Spermatocytic seminoma (T-186._)
Spermatocytoma (T-186._)

9064/3 Germinoma

9070/3 Embryonal carcinoma, NOS
Embryonal adenocarcinoma

9071/3 Endodermal sinus tumor
Yolk sac tumor
Polyvesicular vitelline tumor
Orchioblastoma (T-186._)
Embryonal carcinoma, infantile type

9072/3 Polyembryoma
Embryonal carcinoma, polyembryonal type

9073/1 Gonadoblastoma
Gonocytoma

9080/0 Teratoma, benign
Adult cystic teratoma
Adult teratoma, NOS
Cystic teratoma, NOS
Teratoma, differentiated type
Mature teratoma

9080/1 Teratoma, NOS
Solid teratoma

9080/3 Teratoma, malignant, NOS
Embryonal teratoma
Teratoblastoma, malignant
Immature teratoma

9081/3 Teratocarcinoma
Mixed embryonal carcinoma and teratoma

9082/3 Malignant teratoma, undifferentiated type
Malignant teratoma, anaplastic type

9083/3 Malignant teratoma, intermediate type

9084/0 Dermoid cyst
Dermoid, NOS

9084/3 Dermoid cyst with malignant transformation (T-183.0)

9090/0 Struma ovarii, NOS (T-183.0)

9090/3 Struma ovarii, malignant (T-183.0)

9091/1 Strumal carcinoid (T-183.0)
Struma ovarii and carcinoid (T-183.0)

910 TROPHOBLASTIC NEOPLASMS

9100/0 Hydatidiform mole, NOS (T-181.9)
Hydatid mole (T-181.9)

9100/1 Invasive hydatidiform mole (T-181.9)
Chorioadenoma destruens (T-181.9)
Chorioadenoma (T-181.9)
Invasive mole, NOS (T-181.9)
Malignant hydatidiform mole (T-181.9)

9100/3 Choriocarcinoma
Chorionepithelioma
Chorioepithelioma

9101/3 Choriocarcinoma combined with teratoma
Choriocarcinoma combined with embryonal carcinoma

9102/3 Malignant teratoma, trophoblastic (T-186._)

911 MESONEPHROMAS

9110/0 Mesonephroma, benign
Mesonephric adenoma
Wolffian duct adenoma

9110/1 Mesonephric tumor

9110/3 Mesonephroma, malignant
Mesonephric adenocarcinoma
Mesonephroma, NOS
Mesometanephric carcinoma
Wolffian duct carcinoma

9111/1 Endosalpingioma

912-916 BLOOD VESSEL TUMORS

9120/0 Hemangioma, NOS
  Angioma, NOS
  Chorioangioma (T-181.9)

9120/3 Hemangiosarcoma
  Angiosarcoma

9121/0 Cavernous hemangioma

9122/0 Venous hemangioma

9123/0 Racemose hemangioma
  Arteriovenous hemangioma

9124/3 Kupffer cell sarcoma (T-155.0)

9130/0 Hemangioendothelioma, benign

9130/1 Hemangioendothelioma, NOS
  Angioendothelioma

9130/3 Hemangioendothelioma, malignant
  Hemangioendothelial sarcoma

9131/0 Capillary hemangioma
  Hemangioma simplex
  Infantile hemangioma
  Plexiform hemangioma
  Juvenile hemangioma

9132/0 Intramuscular hemangioma

9140/3 Kaposi's sarcoma
  Multiple hemorrhagic sarcoma

9141/0 Angiokeratoma

9142/0 Verrucous keratotic hemangioma

9150/0 Hemangiopericytoma, benign

9150/1 Hemangiopericytoma, NOS

9150/3 Hemangiopericytoma, malignant

9160/0 Angiofibroma, NOS
  Juvenile angiofibroma (T-147.__)

9161/1 Hemangioblastoma
  Angioblastoma

917 LYMPHATIC VESSEL TUMORS

9170/0 Lymphangioma, NOS
  Lymphangioendothelioma, NOS

9170/3 Lymphangiosarcoma
  Lymphangioendothelial sarcoma
  Lymphangioendothelioma, malignant

9171/0 Capillary lymphangioma

9172/0 Cavernous lymphangioma

9173/0 Cystic lymphangioma
  Hygroma, NOS
  Cystic hygroma

9174/0 Lymphangiomyoma

9174/1 Lymphangiomyomatosis

9175/0 Hemolymphangioma

918-920 OSTEOMAS AND OSTEOSARCOMAS

9180/0 Osteoma, NOS (T-170.__)

9180/3 Osteosarcoma, NOS (T-170.__)
  Osteogenic sarcoma, NOS (T-170.__)
  Osteochondrosarcoma (T-170.__)
  Osteoblastic sarcoma (T-170.__)

9181/3 Chondroblastic osteosarcoma (T-170.__)

9182/3 Fibroblastic osteosarcoma (T-170.__)
  Osteofibrosarcoma (T-170.__)

9183/3 Telangiectatic osteosarcoma (T-170.__)

9184/3 Osteosarcoma in Paget's disease of bone (T-170.__)

9190/3 Juxtacortical osteosarcoma (T-170.__)
  Juxtacortical osteogenic sarcoma (T-170.__)
  Parosteal osteosarcoma (T-170.__)
  Periosteal osteogenic sarcoma (T-170.__)

9191/0 Osteoid osteoma, NOS (T-170.__)

9200/0 Osteoblastoma (T-170._)
    Giant osteoid osteoma (T-170._)

921-924 CHONDROMATOUS NEOPLASMS

9210/0 Osteochondroma (T-170._)
    Cartilaginous exostosis (T-170._)
    Osteocartilaginous exostosis (T-170._)
    Ecchondroma (T-170._)

9210/1 Osteochondromatosis, NOS (T-170._)
    Ecchondrosis (T-170._)

9220/0 Chondroma, NOS (T-170._)
    Enchondroma (T-170._)

9220/1 Chondromatosis, NOS

9220/3 Chondrosarcoma, NOS (T-170._)
    Fibrochondrosarcoma (T-170._)

9221/0 Juxtacortical chondroma (T-170._)
    Periosteal chondroma (T-170._)

9221/3 Juxtacortical chondrosarcoma (T-170._)

9230/0 Chondroblastoma, NOS (T-170._)
    Chondromatous giant cell tumor (T-170._)
    Codman's tumor (T-170._)

9230/3 Chondroblastoma, malignant (T-170._)

9240/3 Mesenchymal chondrosarcoma

9241/0 Chondromyxoid fibroma (T-170._)

925 GIANT CELL TUMORS

9250/1 Giant cell tumor of bone, NOS (T-170._)
    Osteoclastoma, NOS (T-170._)

9250/3 Giant cell tumor of bone, malignant
    (T-170._)
    Osteoclastoma, malignant (T-170._)
    Giant cell sarcoma of bone (T-170._)

9251/1 Giant cell tumor of soft parts, NOS

9251/3 Malignant giant cell tumor of soft parts

926 MISCELLANEOUS BONE TUMORS

9260/3 Ewing's sarcoma (T-170._)
    Ewing's tumor (T-170._)
    Endothelial sarcoma of bone (T-170._)

9261/3 Adamantinoma of long bones (T-170._)
    Tibial adamantinoma (T-170.7)

9262/0 Ossifying fibroma (T-170._)
    Fibro-osteoma (T-170._)
    Osteofibroma (T-170._)

927-934 ODONTOGENIC TUMORS

9270/0 Odontogenic tumor, benign (T-170._)

9270/1 Odontogenic tumor, NOS (T-170._)

9270/3 Odontogenic tumor, malignant (T-170._)
    Odontogenic carcinoma (T-170._)
    Odontogenic sarcoma (T-170._)
    Intraosseous carcinoma (T-170.1)

9271/0 Dentinoma (T-170._)

9272/0 Cementoma, NOS (T-170._)

9273/0 Cementoblastoma, benign (T-170._)

9274/0 Cementifying fibroma (T-170._)

9275/0 Gigantiform cementoma (T-170._)

9280/0 Odontoma, NOS (T-170._)

9281/0 Compound odontoma (T-170._)

9282/0 Complex odontoma (T-170._)

9290/0 Ameloblastic fibro-odontoma (T-170._)
    Fibroameloblastic odontoma (T-170._)

9290/3 Ameloblastic odontosarcoma (T-170._)

9300/0 Adenomatoid odontogenic tumor (T-170._)
    Adenoameloblastoma (T-170._)

9301/0 Calcifying odontogenic cyst (T-170._)

9310/0 Ameloblastoma, NOS (T-170._)
Adamantinoma, NOS *(except of Tibia and Long bones M-9261/3)*(**T-170._**)

9310/3 Ameloblastoma, malignant
Adamantinoma, malignant *(except of Tibia and Long bones M-9261/3)*(**T-170._**)

9311/0 Odontoameloblastoma (T-170._)

9312/0 Squamous odontogenic tumor (T-170._)

9320/0 Odontogenic myxoma (T-170._)
Odontogenic myxofibroma (**T-170._**)

9321/0 Odontogenic fibroma, NOS (T-170._)
Central odontogenic epithelial hamartoma (**T-170._**)
Peripheral odontogenic gingival epithelial hamartoma (**T-170._**)

9330/0 Ameloblastic fibroma (T-170._)

9330/3 Ameloblastic fibrosarcoma (T-170._)
Ameloblastic sarcoma (**T-170._**)
Odontogenic fibrosarcoma (**T-170._**)

9340/0 Calcifying epithelial odontogenic tumor (T-170._)

935-937 MISCELLANEOUS TUMORS

9350/1 Craniopharyngioma (T-194.3)
Rathke's pouch tumor (**T-194.3**)

9360/1 Pinealoma (T-194.4)

9361/1 Pineocytoma (T-194.4)

9362/3 Pineoblastoma (T-194.4)

9363/0 Melanotic neuroectodermal tumor
Retinal anlage tumor
Melanoameloblastoma (**T-170._**)
Melanotic progonoma

9370/3 Chordoma

938-948 GLIOMAS

9380/3 Glioma, malignant (T-191._)
Glioma, NOS *(except Nasal glioma, not neoplastic)* (**T-191._**)
Gliosarcoma (**T-191._**)

9381/3 Gliomatosis cerebri (T-191._)

9382/3 Mixed glioma (T-191._)
Mixed oligo-astrocytoma (**T-191._**)

9383/1 Subependymal glioma (T-191._)
Subependymoma (**T-191._**)
Subependymal astrocytoma, NOS (**T-191._**)

9384/1 Subependymal giant cell astrocytoma (T-191._)

9390/0 Choroid plexus papilloma, NOS (T-191.5)

9390/3 Choroid plexus papilloma, malignant (T-191.5)
Choroid plexus papilloma, anaplastic type (**T-191.5**)

9391/3 Ependymoma, NOS (T-191._)
Epithelial ependymoma (**T-191._**)

9392/3 Ependymoma, anaplastic type (T-191._)
Ependymoblastoma (**T-191._**)

9393/1 Papillary ependymoma (T-191._)

9394/1 Myxopapillary ependymoma (T-191._)

9400/3 Astrocytoma, NOS (T-191._)
Astroglioma (**T-191._**)
Astrocytic glioma (**T-191._**)
Cystic astrocytoma (**T-191._**)

9401/3 Astrocytoma, anaplastic type (T-191._)

9410/3 Protoplasmic astrocytoma (T-191._)

9411/3 Gemistocytic astrocytoma (T-191._)
Gemistocytoma (**T-191._**)

9420/3 Fibrillary astrocytoma (T-191._)
Fibrous astrocytoma (**T-191._**)

9421/3 Pilocytic astrocytoma (T-191._)
    Piloid astrocytoma (T-191._)
    Juvenile astrocytoma (T-191._)

9422/3 Spongioblastoma, NOS (T-191._)

9423/3 Spongioblastoma polare (T-191._)

9430/3 Astroblastoma (T-191._)

9440/3 Glioblastoma, NOS (T-191._)
    Glioblastoma multiforme (T-191._)
    Spongioblastoma multiforme (T-191._)

9441/3 Giant cell glioblastoma (T-191._)

9442/3 Glioblastoma with sarcomatous component
    (T-191._)

9443/3 Primitive polar spongioblastoma (T-191._)

9450/3 Oligodendroglioma, NOS (T-191._)

9451/3 Oligodendroglioma, anaplastic type (T-191._)

9460/3 Oligodendroblastoma (T-191._)

9470/3 Medulloblastoma, NOS (T-191.6)

9471/3 Desmoplastic medulloblastoma (T-191.6)
    Circumscribed arachnoidal cerebellar
      sarcoma (T-191.6)

9472/3 Medullomyoblastoma (T-191.6)

9480/3 Cerebellar sarcoma, NOS (T-191.6)

9481/3 Monstrocellular sarcoma (T-191._)

949-952 NEUROEPITHELIOMATOUS NEOPLASMS

9490/0 Ganglioneuroma
    Gangliocytoma

9490/3 Ganglioneuroblastoma

9491/0 Ganglioneuromatosis

9500/3 Neuroblastoma, NOS
    Sympathicoblastoma
    Sympathicogonioma
    Sympathogonioma

9501/3 Medulloepithelioma, NOS
    Diktyoma

9502/3 Teratoid medulloepithelioma

9503/3 Neuroepithelioma, NOS

9504/3 Spongioneuroblastoma

9505/1 Ganglioglioma
    Glioneuroma
    Neuroastrocytoma

9506/0 Neurocytoma

9507/0 Pacinian tumor

9510/3 Retinoblastoma, NOS (T-190.5)

9511/3 Retinoblastoma, differentiated type (T-190.5)

9512/3 Retinoblastoma, undifferentiated type
    (T-190.5)

9520/3 Olfactory neurogenic tumor

9521/3 Esthesioneurocytoma (T-160._)

9522/3 Esthesioneuroblastoma (T-160._)
    Olfactory neuroblastoma (T-160._)

9523/3 Esthesioneuroepithelioma (T-160._)
    Olfactory neuroepithelioma (T-160._)

953 MENINGIOMAS

9530/0 Meningioma, NOS (T-192._)

9530/1 Meningiomatosis, NOS (T-192._)
    Diffuse meningiomatosis (T-192._)
    Multiple meningiomas (T-192._)

9530/3 Meningioma, malignant (T-192._)
    Leptomeningeal sarcoma (T-192._)
    Meningeal sarcoma (T-192._)
    Meningothelial sarcoma (T-192._)

9531/0 Meningotheliomatous meningioma (T-192._)
Endotheliomatous meningioma (T-192._)
Syncytial meningioma (T-192._)

9532/0 Fibrous meningioma (T-192._)
Fibroblastic meningioma (T-192._)

9533/0 Psammomatous meningioma (T-192._)

9534/0 Angiomatous meningioma (T-192._)

9535/0 Hemangioblastic meningioma (T-192._)
Angioblastic meningioma (T-192._)

9536/0 Hemangiopericytic meningioma (T-192._)

9537/0 Transitional meningioma (T-192._)
Mixed meningioma (T-192._)

9538/1 Papillary meningioma (T-192._)

9539/3 Meningeal sarcomatosis (T-192._)

954-957 NERVE SHEATH TUMORS

9540/0 Neurofibroma, NOS

9540/1 Neurofibromatosis, NOS
Multiple neurofibromatosis
Von Recklinghausen's disease (except of Bone)
Recklinghausen's disease (except of Bone)

9540/3 Neurofibrosarcoma
Neurogenic sarcoma
Neurosarcoma

9541/0 Melanotic neurofibroma

9550/0 Plexiform neurofibroma
Plexiform neuroma

9560/0 Neurilemmoma, NOS
Acoustic neuroma (T-192.0)
Schwannoma, NOS
Neurinoma

9560/1 Neurinomatosis

9560/3 Neurilemmoma, malignant
Schwannoma, malignant
Neurilemmosarcoma

9570/0 Neuroma, NOS

958 GRANULAR CELL TUMORS AND ALVEOLAR SOFT PART SARCOMA

9580/0 Granular cell tumor, NOS
Granular cell myoblastoma, NOS

9580/3 Granular cell tumor, malignant
Granular cell myoblastoma, malignant

9581/3 Alveolar soft part sarcoma

959-963 LYMPHOMAS, NOS OR DIFFUSE

9590/0 Lymphomatous tumor, benign

9590/3 Malignant lymphoma, NOS
Lymphoma, NOS
Malignant lymphoma, diffuse, NOS

9591/3 Malignant lymphoma, non-Hodgkin's type

9600/3 Malignant lymphoma, undifferentiated cell type, NOS
Malignant lymphoma, undifferentiated cell type, non-Burkitt's

9601/3 Malignant lymphoma, stem cell type
Stem cell lymphoma

9602/3 Malignant lymphoma, convoluted cell type, NOS
Malignant lymphoma, lymphoblastic, convoluted cell type

9610/3 Lymphosarcoma, NOS
Lymphosarcoma, diffuse, NOS
Malignant lymphoma, lymphosarcoma type

9611/3 Malignant lymphoma, lymphoplasmacytoid type
Diffuse lymphosarcoma, lymphoplasmacytic
Diffuse lymphosarcoma with plasmacytoid differentiation
Malignant lymphoma, lymphocytic, with plasmacytoid differentiation, diffuse

9612/3 Malignant lymphoma, immunoblastic type
Immunoblastic sarcoma
Immunoblastic lymphosarcoma
Immunoblastic lymphoma

9613/3 Malignant lymphoma, mixed lymphocytic-histiocytic, NOS
Malignant lymphoma, mixed lymphocytic-histiocytic, diffuse
Reticulolymphosarcoma, NOS
Reticulolymphosarcoma, diffuse
Malignant lymphoma, mixed cell type, NOS
Malignant lymphoma, mixed cell type, diffuse
Lymphosarcoma, mixed cell type, NOS
Lymphosarcoma, mixed cell type, diffuse
Malignant lymphoma, mixed small cell and large cell, NOS
Malignant lymphoma, mixed small cell and large cell, diffuse

9614/3 Malignant lymphoma, centroblastic-centrocytic, diffuse
Germinoblastoma, diffuse

9615/3 Malignant lymphoma, follicular center cell, NOS
Malignant lymphoma, follicular center cell, diffuse, NOS

9620/3 Malignant lymphoma, lymphocytic, well differentiated, NOS
Malignant lymphoma, lymphocytic, well differentiated, diffuse
Lymphocytic lymphosarcoma, NOS
Lymphocytic lymphosarcoma, diffuse
Lymphocytic lymphoma, NOS
Lymphocytic lymphoma, diffuse, NOS
Malignant lymphoma, lymphocytic cell type

9621/3 Malignant lymphoma, lymphocytic, intermediate differentiation, NOS
Malignant lymphoma, lymphocytic, intermediate differentiation, diffuse
Lymphocytic lymphosarcoma, intermediate differentiation, NOS
Lymphocytic lymphosarcoma, intermediate differentiation, diffuse

9622/3 Malignant lymphoma, centrocytic
Malignant lymphoma, germinocytic

9623/3 Malignant lymphoma, follicular center cell, cleaved, NOS
Malignant lymphoma, follicular center cell, cleaved, diffuse

9630/3 Malignant lymphoma, lymphocytic, poorly differentiated, NOS
Malignant lymphoma, lymphocytic, poorly differentiated, diffuse
Lymphoblastic lymphosarcoma, NOS
Lymphoblastic lymphosarcoma, diffuse
Lymphocytic lymphoma, poorly differentiated, NOS
Lymphocytic lymphoma, poorly differentiated, diffuse
Lymphoblastoma, NOS
Lymphoblastoma, diffuse
Lymphoblastic lymphoma, NOS
Lymphoblastic lymphoma, diffuse

9631/3 Prolymphocytic lymphosarcoma

9632/3 Malignant lymphoma, centroblastic type, NOS
Malignant lymphoma, centroblastic type, diffuse
Germinoblastic sarcoma, NOS
Germinoblastic sarcoma, diffuse

9633/3 Malignant lymphoma, follicular center cell, non-cleaved, NOS
Malignant lymphoma, follicular center cell, non-cleaved, diffuse

964 RETICULOSARCOMAS

9640/3 Reticulosarcoma, NOS
Malignant lymphoma, histiocytic, NOS
Malignant lymphoma, histiocytic, diffuse
Reticulum cell sarcoma, NOS
Malignant lymphoma, reticulum cell type

9641/3 Reticulosarcoma, pleomorphic cell type
Malignant lymphoma, histiocytic, pleomorphic cell type
Reticulum cell sarcoma, pleomorphic cell type

9642/3 Reticulosarcoma, nodular
Malignant lymphoma, histiocytic, nodular

965-966 HODGKIN'S DISEASE

9650/3 Hodgkin's disease, NOS
Lymphogranuloma, malignant
Lymphogranulomatosis, malignant
Malignant lymphoma, Hodgkin's type

9651/3 Hodgkin's disease, lymphocytic predominance
Hodgkin's disease, lymphocytic-histiocytic
predominance

9652/3 Hodgkin's disease, mixed cellularity

9653/3 Hodgkin's disease, lymphocytic depletion, NOS

9654/3 Hodgkin's disease, lymphocytic depletion, diffuse fibrosis

9655/3 Hodgkin's disease, lymphocytic depletion, reticular type

9656/3 Hodgkin's disease, nodular sclerosis, NOS

9657/3 Hodgkin's disease, nodular sclerosis, cellular phase

9660/3 Hodgkin's paragranuloma

9661/3 Hodgkin's granuloma

9662/3 Hodgkin's sarcoma

969 LYMPHOMAS, NODULAR OR FOLLICULAR

9690/3 Malignant lymphoma, nodular, NOS
Malignant lymphoma, follicular, NOS
Nodular lymphosarcoma, NOS
Follicular lymphosarcoma, NOS
Brill-Symmers's disease
Giant follicular lymphoma
Lymphocytic lymphoma, nodular, NOS

9691/3 Malignant lymphoma, mixed lymphocytic-histiocytic, nodular
Malignant lymphoma, mixed lymphocytic-histiocytic, follicular
Reticulolymphosarcoma, nodular
Reticulolymphosarcoma, follicular
Malignant lymphoma, mixed cell type, nodular
Malignant lymphoma, mixed cell type, follicular
Lymphosarcoma, mixed cell type, nodular
Lymphosarcoma, mixed cell type, follicular
Malignant lymphoma, mixed small cell and large cell, nodular
Malignant lymphoma, mixed small cell and large cell, follicular

9692/3 Malignant lymphoma, centroblastic-centrocytic, follicular
Germinoblastoma, follicular

9693/3 Malignant lymphoma, lymphocytic, well differentiated, nodular
Malignant lymphoma, lymphocytic, well differentiated, follicular
Lymphocytic lymphoma, well differentiated, nodular
Lymphocytic lymphoma, well differentiated, follicular

9694/3 Malignant lymphoma, lymphocytic, intermediate differentiation, nodular
Malignant lymphoma, lymphocytic, intermediate differentiation, follicular
Lymphocytic lymphosarcoma, intermediate differentiation, nodular
Lymphocytic lymphoma, intermediate differentiation, nodular

9695/3 Malignant lymphoma, follicular center cell, cleaved, follicular

9696/3 Malignant lymphoma, lymphocytic, poorly differentiated, nodular
Malignant lymphoma, lymphocytic, poorly differentiated, follicular
Lymphocytic lymphoma, poorly differentiated, nodular
Lymphocytic lymphoma, poorly differentiated, follicular
Lymphoblastic lymphosarcoma, nodular
Lymphoblastic lymphosarcoma, follicular

9697/3 Malignant lymphoma, centroblastic type, follicular
    Germinoblastic sarcoma, follicular

9698/3 Malignant lymphoma, follicular center cell, non-cleaved, follicular

970 MYCOSIS FUNGOIDES

9700/3 Mycosis fungoides

9701/3 Sezary's disease
    Sezary's syndrome

971-972 MISCELLANEOUS RETICULO-ENDOTHELIAL NEOPLASMS

9710/3 Microglioma

9720/3 Malignant histiocytosis
    Malignant reticuloendotheliosis
    Malignant reticulosis

9721/3 Histiocytic medullary reticulosis

9722/3 Letterer-Siwe's disease
    Acute differentiated progressive histiocytosis
    Acute progressive histiocytosis X
    Acute reticulosis of infancy
    Acute infantile reticuloendotheliosis
    Non-lipid reticuloendotheliosis

973 PLASMA CELL TUMORS

9730/3 Plasma cell myeloma
    Plasmacytic myeloma
    Multiple myeloma
    Myeloma, NOS
    Myelomatosis

9731/0 Plasma cell tumor, benign
    Plasmacytoma, benign

9731/1 Plasmacytoma, NOS
    Monostotic myeloma
    Plasma cell tumor, NOS
    Solitary myeloma
    Solitary plasmacytoma

9731/3 Plasma cell tumor, malignant
    Plasma cell sarcoma

974 MAST CELL TUMORS

9740/1 Mastocytoma, NOS
    Mast cell tumor, NOS

9740/3 Mast cell sarcoma
    Malignant mast cell tumor
    Malignant mastocytoma

9741/3 Malignant mastocytosis
    Systemic tissue mast cell disease

975 BURKITT'S TUMOR

9750/3 Burkitt's tumor
    Burkitt's lymphoma
    Malignant lymphoma, undifferentiated, Burkitt's type
    Malignant lymphoma, lymphoblastic, Burkitt's type

980-994 LEUKEMIAS

980 LEUKEMIAS, NOS

9800/3 Leukemia, NOS (T-169._)

9801/3 Acute leukemia, NOS (T-169._)
    Stem cell leukemia (T-169._)
    Blast leukemia (T-169._)
    Blastic leukemia, NOS (T-169._)
    Undifferentiated leukemia (T-169._)

9802/3 Subacute leukemia, NOS (T-169._)

9803/3 Chronic leukemia, NOS (T-169._)

9804/3 Aleukemic leukemia, NOS (T-169._)

981 COMPOUND LEUKEMIAS

9810/3 Compound leukemia (T-169._)
    Mixed leukemia (T-169._)

982 LYMPHOID LEUKEMIAS

9820/3 Lymphoid leukemia, NOS (T-169._)
    Lymphocytic leukemia, NOS (T-169._)
    Lymphatic leukemia, NOS (T-169._)

9821/3 Acute lymphoid leukemia (T-169._)
    Acute lymphocytic leukemia (T-169._)
    Lymphoblastic leukemia (T-169._)
    Acute lymphatic leukemia (T-169._)

9822/3 Subacute lymphoid leukemia (T-169._)
    Subacute lymphocytic leukemia (T-169._)
    Subacute lymphatic leukemia (T-169._)

9823/3 Chronic lymphoid leukemia (T-169._)
    Chronic lymphocytic leukemia (T-169._)
    Chronic lymphatic leukemia (T-169._)

9824/3 Aleukemic lymphoid leukemia (T-169._)
    Aleukemic lymphocytic leukemia (T-169._)
    Aleukemic lymphatic leukemia (T-169._)

9825/3 Prolymphocytic leukemia (T-169._)

983 PLASMA CELL LEUKEMIAS

9830/3 Plasma cell leukemia (T-169._)
    Plasmacytic leukemia (T-169._)

984 ERYTHROLEUKEMIAS

9840/3 Erythroleukemia (T-169._)
    Erythremic myelosis, NOS (T-169._)

9841/3 Acute erythremia (T-169._)
    Di Guglielmo's disease (T-169._)
    Guglielmo's disease (T-169._)
    Acute erythremic myelosis (T-169._)

9842/3 Chronic erythremia (T-169._)

985 LYMPHOSARCOMA CELL LEUKEMIAS

9850/3 Lymphosarcoma cell leukemia (T-169.0)

986 MYELOID LEUKEMIAS

9860/3 Myeloid leukemia, NOS (T-169._)
    Granulocytic leukemia, NOS (T-169._)
    Myelogenous leukemia, NOS (T-169._)
    Myelosis, NOS (T-169._)
    Myelomonocytic leukemia, NOS (T-169._)

9861/3 Acute myeloid leukemia (T-169._)
    Acute granulocytic leukemia (T-169._)
    Blastic granulocytic leukemia (T-169._)
    Acute myelogenous leukemia (T-169._)
    Myeloblastic leukemia (T-169._)
    Acute myelocytic leukemia (T-169._)
    Acute myelomonocytic leukemia (T-169._)
    Acute myelosis, NOS (T-169._)

9862/3 Subacute myeloid leukemia (T-169._)
    Subacute granulocytic leukemia (T-169._)
    Subacute myelogenous leukemia (T-169._)
    Subacute myelosis (T-169._)

9863/3 Chronic myeloid leukemia (T-169._)
    Chronic granulocytic leukemia (T-169._)
    Myelocytic leukemia, NOS (T-169._)
    Chronic myelogenous leukemia (T-169._)
    Chronic myelomonocytic leukemia (T-169._)
    Naegeli-type monocytic leukemia (T-169._)
    Chronic myelosis (T-169._)

9864/3 Aleukemic myeloid leukemia (T-169._)
    Aleukemic granulocytic leukemia (T-169._)
    Aleukemic myelogenous leukemia (T-169._)
    Aleukemic myelosis (T-169._)

9865/3 Neutrophilic leukemia (T-169._)

9866/3 Acute promyelocytic leukemia (T-169._)

987 BASOPHILIC LEUKEMIAS

9870/3 Basophilic leukemia (T-169._)

988 EOSINOPHILIC LEUKEMIAS

9880/3 Eosinophilic leukemia (T-169._)

989 MONOCYTIC LEUKEMIAS

9890/3 Monocytic leukemia, NOS (T-169._)
    Histiocytic leukemia (T-169._)
    Schilling-type monocytic leukemia (T-169._)
    Monocytoid leukemia, NOS (T-169._)

9891/3 Acute monocytic leukemia (T-169._)
    Acute monocytoid leukemia (T-169._)
    Monoblastic leukemia (T-169._)

9892/3 Subacute monocytic leukemia (T-169._)
    Subacute monocytoid leukemia (T-169._)

9893/3 Chronic monocytic leukemia (T-169._)
    Chronic monocytoid leukemia (T-169._)

9894/3 Aleukemic monocytic leukemia (T-169._)
    Aleukemic monocytoid leukemia (T-169._)

990-994 MISCELLANEOUS LEUKEMIAS

9900/3 Mast cell leukemia (T-169._)

9910/3 Megakaryocytic leukemia (T-169._)
    Megakaryocytoid leukemia (T-169._)
    Thrombocytic leukemia (T-169._)

9920/3 Megakaryocytic myelosis (T-169._)

9930/3 Myeloid sarcoma
    Chloroma
    Granulocytic sarcoma
    Myelosarcoma

9940/3 Hairy cell leukemia (T-169._)
    Leukemic reticuloendotheliosis

995-997 MISCELLANEOUS MYELO-PROLIFERATIVE AND LYMPHO-PROLIFERATIVE DISORDERS

9950/1 Polycythemia vera (T-169._)
    Polycythemia rubra vera (T-169._)

9951/1 Acute panmyelosis (T-169.1)

9960/1 Chronic myeloproliferative disease (T-169._)

9961/1 Myelosclerosis with myeloid metaplasia (T-169.1)
    Megakaryocytic myelosclerosis (T-169.1)

9962/1 Idiopathic thrombocythemia (T-169._)

9970/1 Chronic lymphoproliferative disease

999 NO MICROSCOPIC CONFIRMATION OF TUMOR

9990/0 No microscopic confirmation; clinically benign tumor

9990/1 No microscopic confirmation; clinically tumor, NOS

9990/3 No microscopic confirmation; clinically malignant tumor *(cancer)*

9990/6 No microscopic confirmation; clinically metastatic tumor *(cancer)*

ALPHABETIC INDEX

M------- Not neoplastic; See Introduction page *xx*.

NOS - Not Otherwise Specified; See Introduction page *vi*.

- A -

Abdomen
T-195.2   NOS
T-171.5   connective tissue
T-171.5   muscle
T-173.5   skin
T-171.5   subcutaneous tissue

M-8822/1 Abdominal desmoid
M-8822/1 Abdominal fibromatosis

Abdominal
T-171.5   aorta
T-150.2   esophagus
T-196.2   lymph node
T-171.5   vena cava

Abdominal wall
T-195.2   NOS
T-173.5   NOS (carcinoma, melanoma, nevus)
T-171.5   NOS (sarcoma, lipoma)
T-171.5   adipose tissue
T-171.5   connective tissue
T-171.5   fatty tissue
T-171.5   fibrous tissue
T-171.5   muscle
T-171.5   skeletal muscle
T-173.5   skin
T-171.5   soft tissue
T-171.5   subcutaneous tissue

T-192.0   Abducens nerve

M------- Acanthoma, clear cell *(SNOMED M-72530)*
M------- Acanthosis nigricans *(SNOMED M-57330)*

Accessory
T-160.9   nasal sinus
T-192.0   nerve, NOS
T-192.0   nerve, spinal
T-160.9   sinus, NOS
T-160.9   sinus, nasal

T-170.6   Acetabulum

M-8730/0 Achromic nevus (T-173._)

Acidophil
M-8280/3   adenocarcinoma (T-194.3)
M-8280/0   adenoma (T-194.3)
M-8280/3   carcinoma (T-194.3)

M-8281/0 Acidophil-basophil adenoma, mixed (T-194.3)
M-8281/3 Acidophil-basophil carcinoma, mixed (T-194.3)

Acinar
M-8550/3   adenocarcinoma
M-8550/0   adenoma
M-8550/3   carcinoma

Acinar cell
M-8550/0   adenoma
M-8550/3   carcinoma
M-8550/1   tumor

Acinic cell
M-8550/3   adenocarcinoma
M-8550/0   adenoma
M-8550/1   tumor

T-192.0   Acoustic nerve

M-9560/0 Acoustic neuroma (T-192.0)

T-170.4   Acromioclavicular joint

M-8402/0 Acrospiroma, eccrine (T-173._)
M------- Actinic keratosis *(SNOMED M-72850)*

Acute

M-9722/3 differentiated progressive histiocytosis
M-9841/3 erythremia (T-169._)
M-9841/3 erythremic myelosis (T-169._)
M-9722/3 infantile reticuloendotheliosis
M-9861/3 myelosis, NOS (T-169._)
M-9951/1 panmyelosis (T-169.1)
M-9722/3 progressive histiocytosis X
M-9722/3 reticulosis of infancy

Adamantinoma

M-9310/0 NOS *(except of Tibia and Long bones M-9261/3)*(T-170._)
M-9261/3 long bones (T-170._)
M-9310/3 malignant *(except of Tibia and Long bones M-9261/3)*(T-170._)
M-9261/3 tibial (T-170.7)

M-8570/3 Adenoacanthoma
M-9300/0 Adenoameloblastoma (T-170._)

Adenocarcinoma *(see also Carcinoma)*

M-8140/3 NOS
M-8140/6 NOS, metastatic
M-8280/3 acidophil (T-194.3)
M-8550/3 acinar
M-8550/3 acinic cell
M-8370/3 adrenal cortical (T-194.0)
M-8251/3 alveolar
M-8560/3 and epidermoid carcinoma, mixed
M-8560/3 and squamous cell carcinoma, mixed
M-8401/3 apocrine
M-8300/3 basophil (T-194.3)
M-8160/3 bile duct (T-155._)
M-8250/3 bronchiolar (T-162._)
M-8250/3 bronchiolo-alveolar (T-162._)
M-8420/3 ceruminous (T-173.2)
M-8270/3 chromophobe (T-194.3)
M-8310/3 clear cell, NOS
M-8310/3 clear cell, mesonephroid type
M-8480/3 colloid
M-8200/3 cylindroid type
M-8145/3 diffuse type (T-151._)
M-8500/3 duct, NOS
M-8500/3 duct, infiltrating (T-174._)
M-9070/3 embryonal
M-8380/3 endometrioid
M-8280/3 eosinophil (T-194.3)

Adenocarcinoma (Cont'd)

M-8330/3 follicular, NOS (T-193.9)
M-8332/3 follicular, moderately differentiated type (T-193.9)
M-8331/3 follicular, pure follicle type (T-193.9)
M-8332/3 follicular, trabecular type (T-193.9)
M-8331/3 follicular, well differentiated type (T-193.9)
M-8340/3 follicular and papillary (T-193.9)
M-8480/3 gelatinous
M-8320/3 granular cell
M-8290/3 Hürthle cell (T-193.9)
M-8140/2 in-situ
M-8210/3 in adenomatous polyp
M-8220/3 in adenomatous polyposis coli (T-153._)
M-8210/3 in polypoid adenoma
M-8210/3 in tubular adenoma
M-8261/3 in villous adenoma
M-8500/3 infiltrating duct (T-174._)
M-8530/3 inflammatory (T-174._)
M-8144/3 intestinal type (T-151._)
M-8500/2 intraductal, non-infiltrating, NOS
M-8503/2 intraductal, non-infiltrating, papillary
M-8150/3 islet cell (T-157._)
M-8154/3 islet cell and exocrine, mixed (T-157._)
M-8520/3 lobular (T-174._)
M-8510/3 medullary
M-9110/3 mesonephric
M-8310/3 mesonephroid type, clear cell
M-8323/3 mixed cell
M-8480/3 mucinous
M-8481/3 mucin-producing
M-8481/3 mucin-secreting
M-8480/3 mucoid
M-8300/3 mucoid cell (T-194.3)
M-8480/3 mucous
M-8500/2 non-infiltrating, intraductal, NOS
M-8503/2 non-infiltrating, intraductal, papillary
M-8350/3 nonencapsulated sclerosing (T-193.9)
M-8290/3 oncocytic
M-8290/3 oxyphilic
M-8260/3 papillary, NOS
M-8340/3 papillary and follicular (T-193.9)
M-8503/2 papillary, intraductal, non-infiltrating
M-8460/3 papillary, serous (T-183.0)
M-8450/3 papillocystic
M-8470/3 pseudomucinous (T-183.0)

Adenoma (Cont'd)

M-8210/0	polypoid
M-8210/3	polypoid, adenocarcinoma in
M-8410/0	sebaceous (T-173._)
M-------	sebaceum *(SNOMED M-75730)*
M-8640/0	Sertoli cell
M-8390/0	skin appendage (T-173._)
M-8400/0	sweat gland (T-173._)
M-8640/0	testicular
M-8190/0	trabecular
M-8211/0	tubular, NOS
M-8210/3	tubular, adenocarcinoma in
M-8640/0	tubular, Pick's
M-8263/0	tubulovillous
M-8263/0	villoglandular
M-8261/1	villous, NOS
M-8261/3	villous, adenocarcinoma in
M-8322/0	water-clear cell (T-194.1)
M-9110/0	Wolffian duct

M-8360/1 Adenomas, multiple, endocrine
M-9054/0 Adenomatoid tumor, NOS
M-9300/0 Adenomatoid tumor, odontogenic (T-170._)

Adenomatosis

M-8220/0	NOS (T-153._)
M-8360/1	endocrine
M-------	fibrosing *(SNOMED M-74220)*
M-8506/0	nipple, erosive (T-174.0)
M-8250/1	pulmonary (T-162._)

Adenomatous

M-------	goiter *(SNOMED M-71640)*
M-------	hyperplasia *(SNOMED M-72420)*
M-8210/0	polyp, NOS
M-8210/3	polyp, adenocarcinoma in
M-8210/3	polyp, carcinoma in
M-8220/0	polyposis coli (T-153._)
M-8220/3	polyposis coli, adenocarcinoma in (T-153._)
M-8221/0	polyps, multiple

M-8932/0 Adenomyoma
M------- Adenomyomatous hyperplasia
  (SNOMED M-72440)
M------- Adenomyosis, NOS *(SNOMED M-76510)*
M-8960/3 Adenosarcoma (T-189.0)

Adenosis

M-------	NOS *(SNOMED M-74200)*
M-------	fibrosing *(SNOMED M-74220)*
M-------	florid *(SNOMED M-74260)*
M-------	sclerosing *(SNOMED M-74220)*

M-8560/3 Adenosquamous carcinoma

Adipose tissue

T-171.9	NOS
T-171.5	abdominal wall
T-171.2	antecubital space
T-171.2	arm
T-171.4	axilla
T-171.7	back
T-171.6	buttock
T-171.3	calf
T-171.0	cervical region
T-171.0	cheek
T-171.4	chest wall
T-171.0	face
T-171.7	flank
T-171.3	foot
T-171.2	forearm
T-171.6	gluteal region
T-171.6	groin
T-171.2	hand
T-171.0	head
T-171.3	hip
T-171.4	infraclavicular region
T-171.6	inguinal region
T-171.3	knee
T-171.3	leg
T-171.0	neck
T-171.3	popliteal space
T-171.6	sacrococcygeal region
T-171.0	scalp
T-171.4	scapular region
T-171.2	shoulder
T-171.0	supraclavicular region
T-171.0	temple
T-171.3	thigh
T-171.4	thoracic wall
T-171.7	trunk

T-183.9 Adnexa, NOS
T-183.9 Adnexa, uterine

M-8390/3 Adnexal carcinoma (T-173._)
M-8390/0 Adnexal tumor (T-173._)

Adrenal

T-194.0	NOS
T-194.0	cortex
T-194.0	gland
T-194.0	medulla

M-8370/3 Adrenal cortical adenocarcinoma (T-194.0)

Adrenal cortical adenoma

M-8370/0	NOS (T-194.0)
M-8373/0	clear cell type (T-194.0)
M-8371/0	compact cell type (T-194.0)
M-8374/0	glomerulosa cell type (T-194.0)
M-8372/0	heavily pigmented variant (T-194.0)
M-8375/0	mixed cell type (T-194.0)

M-8370/3 Adrenal cortical carcinoma (T-194.0)

Adrenal cortical tumor

M-8370/0	NOS (T-194.0)
M-8370/0	benign (T-194.0)
M-8370/3	malignant (T-194.0)

M-8671/0 Adrenal rest tumor

Adult

M-8904/0	rhabdomyoma
M-9080/0	teratoma, NOS
M-9080/0	teratoma, cystic

M-8821/1 Aggressive fibromatosis

T-173.3	Ala nasi
T-159.9	Alimentary tract, NOS

M-8152/0 Alpha-cell adenoma (T-157._)
M-8152/3 Alpha-cell tumor, malignant (T-157._)

Alveolar

M-8251/3	adenocarcinoma
M-8251/0	adenoma
M-8251/3	carcinoma
M-8920/3	rhabdomyosarcoma
M-9581/3	soft part sarcoma

M-8250/3 Alveolar cell carcinoma (T-162._)

Alveolar mucosa

T-143.9	NOS
T-143.1	lower
T-143.0	upper

Alveolar ridge mucosa

T-143.9	NOS
T-143.1	lower
T-143.0	upper

T-145.1 Alveolar sulcus

Alveolus

T-143.9	NOS
T-143.1	lower
T-143.0	upper

M-8730/3 Amelanotic melanoma

Ameloblastic

M-9290/0	fibro-odontoma (T-170._)
M-9330/0	fibroma (T-170._)
M-9330/3	fibrosarcoma (T-170._)
M-9290/3	odontosarcoma (T-170._)
M-9330/3	sarcoma (T-170._)

M-9310/0 Ameloblastoma, NOS (T-170._)
M-9310/3 Ameloblastoma, malignant (T-170._)

T-156.2	Ampulla of Vater
T-154.1	Ampulla, rectal

M------- Amputation neuroma (SNOMED M-49770)
M------- Amyloid tumor (SNOMED M-55160)

T-154.2	Anal canal
T-154.2	Anal sphincter

M-___/_(4) Anaplastic (see Grading code, page 20)

Anaplastic type

M-9401/3	astrocytoma (T-191._)
M-8021/3	carcinoma, NOS
M-9390/3	choroid plexus papilloma (T-191.5)
M-9392/3	ependymoma (T-191._)
M-9082/3	malignant teratoma
M-9451/3	oligodendroglioma (T-191._)
M-9062/3	seminoma (T-186._)

Androblastoma

M-8630/1	NOS
M-8630/0	benign
M-8630/3	malignant
M-8640/0	tubular, NOS
M-8641/0	tubular with lipid storage (T-183.0)

M------- Aneurysmal bone cyst (SNOMED M-33640)
M-9535/0 Angioblastic meningioma (T-192._)
M-9161/1 Angioblastoma
M-9130/1 Angioendothelioma
M-9160/0 Angiofibroma, NOS
M-9160/0 Angiofibroma, juvenile (T-147._)
M------- Angiofollicular hyperplasia, benign
(SNOMED M-72260)
M------- Angio-immunoblastic lymphadenopathy
(SNOMED M-72280)

M-9141/0 Angiokeratoma

M-8894/0 Angioleiomyoma

M-8861/0 Angiolipoma, NOS

M-8861/1 Angiolipoma, infiltrating

M-9120/0 Angioma, NOS

M------- Angioma, spider *(SNOMED M-76330)*

M------- Angiomatosis, NOS *(SNOMED M-76310)*

M------- Angiomatous lymphoid hamartoma
           (SNOMED M-72260)

M-9534/0 Angiomatous meningioma (T-192._)

M-8860/0 Angiomyolipoma

M-8860/3 Angiomyoliposarcoma

M-8894/0 Angiomyoma

M-8894/3 Angiomyosarcoma

M-9120/3 Angiosarcoma

Ankle

T-195.5 NOS

T-173.7 NOS (carcinoma, melanoma, nevus)

T-171.3 NOS (sarcoma, lipoma)

T-170.8 bone

T-171.3 connective tissue

T-171.3 fibrous tissue

T-170.8 joint

T-173.7 skin

T-171.3 soft tissue

T-171.3 subcutaneous tissue

T-171.3 tendon

T-171.3 tendon sheath

T-154.8 Anorectal junction

T-154.8 Anorectum

Antecubital space

T-195.4 NOS

T-173.6 NOS (carcinoma, melanoma, nevus)

T-171.2 NOS (sarcoma, lipoma)

T-171.2 adipose tissue

T-171.2 connective tissue

T-171.2 fatty tissue

T-171.2 fibrous tissue

T-173.6 skin

T-171.2 soft tissue

T-171.2 subcutaneous tissue

Anterior

T-191.9 cranial fossa

T-144.0 floor of mouth

T-164.2 mediastinum

T-146.4 surface of epiglottis

Anterior tongue

T-141.4 NOS

T-141.1 dorsal surface

T-141.3 ventral surface

Anterior 2/3 of tongue

T-141.4 NOS

T-141.1 dorsal surface

T-141.3 ventral surface

Anterior wall

T-147.3 nasopharynx

T-151.8 stomach, NOS *(not classifiable to T-151.0 to T-151.4)*

T-188.3 urinary bladder

Antrum

T-160.2 NOS

T-151.2 gastric

T-160.1 mastoid

T-160.2 maxillary

T-151.2 pyloric

T-151.2 stomach

T-154.3 Anus, NOS *(excludes Skin of anus and Perianal skin T-173.5)*

T-173.5 Anus, skin

T-171.4 Aorta, NOS

T-171.5 Aorta, abdominal

T-194.6 Aortic body

M-8691/1 Aortic body paraganglioma (T-194.6)

M-8691/1 Aortic body tumor (T-194.6)

T-196.2 Aortic lymph node

M-8401/3 Apocrine adenocarcinoma

M-8401/0 Apocrine adenoma

Aponeurosis

T-171.9 NOS

T-171.2 palmar

T-171.3 plantar

M------- Aponeurotic fibroma, juvenile
           (SNOMED M-76150)

T-153.5 Appendix

Arachnoid
T-192.1   NOS
T-192.1   intracranial
T-192.3   spinal

T-174.0   Areola

M-8241/1   Argentaffin carcinoid tumor, NOS
M-8241/3   Argentaffin carcinoid tumor, malignant
M-8241/1   Argentaffinoma, NOS
M-8241/3   Argentaffinoma, malignant

Arm
T-195.4   NOS
T-173.6   NOS (carcinoma, melanoma, nevus)
T-171.2   NOS (sarcoma, lipoma)
T-171.2   adipose tissue
T-170.4   bone
T-171.2   connective tissue
T-171.2   fatty tissue
T-171.2   fibrous tissue
T-196.3   lymph node
T-171.2   muscle
T-171.2   skeletal muscle
T-173.6   skin
T-171.2   soft tissue
T-171.2   subcutaneous tissue
T-171.2   tendon
T-171.2   tendon sheath

Arrhenoblastoma
M-8630/1   NOS
M-8630/0   benign
M-8630/3   malignant

M-9123/0   Arteriovenous hemangioma

Artery
T-171.9   NOS
T-171.4   aorta, NOS
T-171.5   aorta, abdominal
T-171.4   axillary
T-171.0   carotid
T-171.5   celiac
T-171.3   femoral
T-171.6   iliac
T-171.4   internal mammary
T-171.5   mesenteric
T-171.2   radial
T-171.5   renal
T-171.4   subclavian
T-171.2   ulnar

T-170.9   Articular cartilage, NOS

Aryepiglottic fold
T-148.2   NOS (excludes Laryngeal aspect of
           aryepiglottic fold T-161.1)
T-148.2   hypopharyngeal aspect
T-161.1   laryngeal aspect

T-161.3   Arytenoid cartilage
T-148.2   Arytenoid fold
T-153.6   Ascending colon

M-9430/3   Astroblastoma (T-191._)
M-9400/3   Astrocytic glioma (T-191._)

Astrocytoma
M-9400/3   NOS (T-191._)
M-9401/3   anaplastic type (T-191._)
M-9400/3   cystic (T-191._)
M-9420/3   fibrillary (T-191._)
M-9420/3   fibrous (T-191._)
M-9411/3   gemistocytic (T-191._)
M-9421/3   juvenile (T-191._)
M-9421/3   pilocytic (T-191._)
M-9421/3   piloid (T-191._)
M-9410/3   protoplasmic (T-191._)
M-9383/1   subependymal, NOS (T-191._)
M-9384/1   subependymal giant cell (T-191._)

M-9400/3   Astroglioma (T-191._)

T-170.2   Atlas
T-164.1   Atrium, cardiac

M-------   Atrophy-associated hyperplasia
           (SNOMED M-72425)

Atypical
M-8830/1   fibrous histiocytoma
M-8831/1   fibroxanthoma
M-------   hyperplasia (SNOMED M-72005)

Auditory
T-173.2   canal, NOS
T-173.2   canal, external
T-173.2   meatus, external
T-160.1   tube

T-173.2   Auricle, NOS
T-173.2   Auricle, skin

Auricular

T-173.2	canal, NOS
T-173.2	canal, external
T-171.0	cartilage
T-196.0	lymph node

T-171.9   Autonomic nervous system

Axilla

T-195.1	NOS
T-173.5	NOS (carcinoma, melanoma, nevus)
T-171.4	NOS (sarcoma, lipoma)
T-171.4	adipose tissue
T-171.4	connective tissue
T-171.4	fatty tissue
T-171.4	fibrous tissue
T-196.3	lymph node
T-173.5	skin
T-171.4	soft tissue
T-171.4	subcutaneous tissue

Axillary

T-171.4	artery
T-196.3	lymph node
T-174.6	tail of breast

T-170.2   Axis

- B -

Back

T-195.8	NOS
T-173.5	NOS (carcinoma, melanoma, nevus)
T-171.7	NOS (sarcoma, lipoma)
T-171.7	adipose tissue
T-170.2	bone
T-171.7	connective tissue
T-171.7	fascia
T-171.7	fatty tissue
T-171.7	fibrous tissue
T-171.7	muscle
T-171.7	skeletal muscle
T-173.5	skin
T-171.7	soft tissue
T-171.7	subcutaneous tissue
T-171.7	tendon
T-171.7	tendon sheath

M-8722/3	Balloon cell melanoma
M-8722/0	Balloon cell nevus (T-173._)

T-184.1   Bartholin's gland

Basal cell

M-8147/0	adenoma
M-8090/3	carcinoma, NOS (T-173._)
M-8093/3	carcinoma, fibroepithelial type (T-173._)
M-8092/3	carcinoma, morphea type (T-173._)
M-8091/3	carcinoma, multicentric (T-173._)
M-8090/3	carcinoma, pigmented (T-173._)
M-8090/3	epithelioma (T-173._)
M-------	papilloma (SNOMED M-72750)
M-8090/1	tumor (T-173._)

T-191.0   Basal ganglia

M-8094/3	Basal-squamous cell carcinoma, mixed (T-173._)
M-8123/3	Basaloid carcinoma

T-141.0	Base of tongue, NOS
T-141.0	Base of tongue, dorsal surface
T-191.7	Basis pedunculi

Basophil

M-8281/0	acidophil adenoma, mixed (T-194.3)
M-8281/3	acidophil carcinoma, mixed (T-194.3)
M-8300/3	adenocarcinoma (T-194.3)
M-8300/0	adenoma (T-194.3)
M-8300/3	carcinoma (T-194.3)

M-8094/3	Basosquamous carcinoma (T-173._)
M-------	Basosquamous papilloma (SNOMED M-72750)
M-____/0	Benign (see Behavior code, page 20)
M-8151/0	Beta-cell adenoma (T-157._)
M-8151/3	Beta-cell tumor, malignant (T-157._)

T-171.2	Biceps brachii muscle
T-171.3	Biceps femoris muscle

Bile duct

M-8160/3	adenocarcinoma (T-155._)
M-8160/0	adenoma (T-155._)
M-8160/3	carcinoma (T-155._)
M-8180/3	carcinoma and hepatocellular carcinoma, mixed (T-155.0)
M-8161/3	cystadenocarcinoma (T-155._)
M-8161/0	cystadenoma (T-155._)

Bile duct

T-156.1	NOS
T-156.1	common
T-156.1	cystic
T-156.1	extrahepatic
T-156.1	hepatic
T-155.1	intrahepatic

Biliary

T-155.1	canaliculus
T-156.1	duct, NOS
T-156.9	tract, NOS

M-------	Birthmark *(SNOMED M-75540)*
M-8893/0	Bizarre leiomyoma
M-8372/0	Black adenoma **(T-194.0)**

T-188.9	Bladder, NOS

Bladder, urinary

T-188.9	NOS
T-188.3	anterior wall
T-188.1	dome
T-188.5	internal urethral orifice
T-188.2	lateral wall
T-188.5	neck
T-188.4	posterior wall
T-188.0	trigone
T-188.7	urachus
T-188.6	ureteric orifice
T-188.9	wall, NOS
T-188.3	wall, anterior
T-188.2	wall, lateral
T-188.4	wall, posterior

T-169.0	Blood
T-171.9	Blood vessel, NOS

Blue nevus

M-8780/0	NOS **(T-173._)**
M-8790/0	cellular **(T-173._)**
M-8790/0	giant **(T-173._)**
M-8780/0	Jadassohn's **(T-173._)**
M-8780/3	malignant **(T-173._)**

Body

T-194.6	aortic
T-194.5	carotid
T-190.0	ciliary

Body (Cont'd)

T-194.6	coccygeal
T-157.1	pancreas
T-194.6	para-aortic
T-187.3	penis
T-151.4	stomach
T-182.0	uterus

Bone

T-170.9	NOS
T-170.6	acetabulum
T-170.8	ankle
T-170.4	arm
T-170.2	atlas
T-170.2	axis
T-170.2	back
T-170.0	calvarium
T-170.5	carpal
T-170.3	clavicle
T-170.6	coccyx
T-170.0	cranial
T-170.0	ethmoid
T-170.0	face *(excludes Mandible T-170.1)*
T-170.0	facial
T-170.7	femur
T-170.7	fibula
T-170.5	finger
T-170.8	foot
T-170.4	forearm
T-170.0	frontal
T-170.5	hand
T-170.8	heel
T-170.6	hip
T-170.4	humerus
T-170.0	hyoid
T-170.6	ilium
T-170.6	innominate
T-170.6	ischium
T-170.1	jaw, NOS
T-170.1	jaw, lower
T-170.0	jaw, upper
T-170.7	leg
T-170.7	long, lower limb
T-170.4	long, upper limb
T-170.1	lower jaw
T-170.7	lower limb, long
T-170.8	lower limb, short
T-170.1	mandible
T-169.1	marrow
T-170.0	maxilla

Bone (Cont'd)

T-170.5	metacarpal
T-170.8	metatarsal
T-170.0	nasal
T-170.0	occipital
T-170.0	orbital
T-170.0	parietal
T-170.8	patella
T-170.6	pelvic
T-170.8	phalanx of foot
T-170.5	phalanx of hand
T-170.6	pubic
T-170.4	radius
T-170.3	rib
T-170.6	sacrum
T-170.4	scapula
T-170.8	short, lower limb
T-170.5	short, upper limb
T-170.4	shoulder
T-170.4	shoulder girdle
T-170.9	skeletal
T-170.0	skull
T-170.0	sphenoid
T-170.2	spinal column
T-170.2	spine
T-170.3	sternum
T-170.8	tarsal
T-170.0	temporal
T-170.5	thumb
T-170.7	tibia
T-170.8	toe
T-170.4	ulna
T-170.0	upper jaw
T-170.4	upper limb, long
T-170.5	upper limb, short
T-170.2	vertebra
T-170.2	vertebral column (excludes Sacrum and Coccyx T-170.6)
T-170.5	wrist
T-170.0	zygomatic

T-141.2	Border of tongue
M-____/1	Borderline malignancy (see Behavior code, page 20)
M-8910/3	Botryoid sarcoma

Bowel

T-159.0	NOS
T-153.9	large
T-152.9	small

M-8081/2	Bowen's disease (T-173._)
M-8081/2	Bowen's type intraepidermal squamous cell carcinoma (T-173._)

Brachial

T-196.3	lymph node
T-171.2	nerve
T-171.2	plexus
T-171.2	Brachialis muscle

Brain

T-191.9	NOS
T-192.1	arachnoid, NOS
T-191.0	basal ganglia
T-191.7	basis pedunculi
T-191.0	capsule, internal
T-191.0	central white matter
T-191.6	cerebellopontine angle
T-191.6	cerebellum, NOS
T-191.6	cerebellum, vermis
T-191.0	cerebral cortex
T-191.0	cerebral hemisphere
T-192.1	cerebral meninges
T-191.7	cerebral peduncle
T-191.5	cerebral ventricle
T-191.0	cerebral white matter
T-191.0	cerebrum
T-192.0	chiasm, optic
T-191.5	choroid plexus
T-191.8	corpus callosum
T-191.0	corpus striatum
T-191.0	cortex, cerebral
T-192.1	cranial dura mater
T-192.1	cranial meninges
T-192.1	cranial pia mater
T-192.1	dura, NOS
T-192.1	dura mater, NOS
T-192.1	dura mater, cranial
T-191.5	ependyma
T-192.1	falx, NOS
T-192.1	falx cerebelli
T-192.1	falx cerebri
T-191.5	fourth ventricle
T-191.1	frontal lobe
T-191.1	frontal pole
T-191.0	ganglia, basal
T-191.0	globus pallidus
T-191.0	hemisphere, cerebral
T-191.2	hippocampus
T-191.0	hypothalamus
T-191.0	insula

Brain (Cont'd)

T-191.0	internal capsule
T-192.1	intracranial arachnoid
T-192.1	intracranial meninges
T-191.0	island of Reil
T-191.5	lateral ventricle
T-191.1	lobe, frontal
T-191.4	lobe, occipital
T-191.3	lobe, parietal
T-191.2	lobe, temporal
T-191.7	medulla oblongata
T-192.1	meninges, NOS
T-192.1	meninges, cerebral
T-191.7	midbrain
T-191.4	occipital lobe
T-191.4	occipital pole
T-191.7	olive
T-191.0	operculum
T-192.0	optic chiasm
T-192.0	optic tract
T-191.0	pallium
T-191.3	parietal lobe
T-191.7	peduncle, cerebral
T-192.1	pia mater, NOS
T-191.5	plexus, choroid
T-191.1	pole, frontal
T-191.4	pole, occipital
T-191.7	pons
T-191.0	putamen
T-191.7	pyramid
T-191.0	rhinencephalon
T-191.7	stem
T-191.8	tapetum
T-191.2	temporal lobe
T-192.1	tentorium, NOS
T-192.1	tentorium cerebelli
T-191.0	thalamus
T-191.5	third ventricle
T-192.0	tract, optic
T-191.2	uncus
T-191.5	ventricle, NOS
T-191.5	ventricle, cerebral
T-191.5	ventricle, fourth
T-191.5	ventricle, lateral
T-191.5	ventricle, third
T-191.6	vermis, cerebellum
T-191.0	white matter, central
T-191.0	white matter, cerebral

T-146.8	Branchial cleft *(site of neoplasm)*

Breast, female

T-174.9	NOS *(excludes Skin of breast T-173.5)*
T-174.0	areola
T-174.6	axillary tail
T-174.1	central portion
T-174.8	inner
T-174.8	lower
T-174.3	lower-inner quadrant
T-174.5	lower-outer quadrant
T-174.8	midline
T-174.0	nipple
T-174.8	outer
T-174.3	quadrant, lower-inner
T-174.5	quadrant, lower-outer
T-174.2	quadrant, upper-inner
T-174.4	quadrant, upper-outer
T-173.5	skin
T-174.6	tail
T-174.8	upper
T-174.2	upper-inner quadrant
T-174.4	upper-outer quadrant

T-175.9	Breast, male, NOS *(excludes Skin of breast T-173.5)*

T-173.5	Breast, skin

Brenner tumor

M-9000/0	NOS (T-183.0)
M-9000/1	borderline malignancy (T-183.0)
M-9000/3	malignant (T-183.0)
M-9000/1	proliferating (T-183.0)

M-9690/3	Brill-Symmers's disease

T-183.3	Broad ligament

Bronchial adenoma

M-8140/1	NOS (T-162._)
M-8240/3	carcinoid type (T-162._)
M-8200/3	cylindroid type (T-162._)

T-196.1	Bronchial lymph node

M-8250/3	Bronchiolar adenocarcinoma (T-162._)
M-8250/3	Bronchiolar carcinoma (T-162._)

T-162.9	Bronchiole

M-8250/3	Bronchiolo-alveolar adenocarcinoma (T-162._)
M-8250/3	Bronchiolo-alveolar carcinoma (T-162._)

T-162.9 Bronchogenic
T-196.1 Bronchopulmonary lymph node

Bronchus
T-162.9 NOS
T-162.2 carina
T-162.5 lower lobe
T-162.2 main
T-162.4 middle lobe
T-162.3 upper lobe

M-8100/0 Brooke's tumor (T-173._)

T-173.3 Brow

M-8880/0 Brown fat tumor

Buccal
T-145.9 cavity
T-145.0 mucosa
T-145.1 sulcus

M-9750/3 Burkitt's lymphoma
M-9750/3 Burkitt's tumor

T-171.9 Bursa, NOS

Buttock
T-195.3 NOS
T-173.5 NOS (carcinoma, melanoma, nevus)
T-171.6 NOS (sarcoma, lipoma)
T-171.6 adipose tissue
T-171.6 connective tissue
T-171.6 fatty tissue
T-171.6 fibrous tissue
T-171.6 muscle
T-171.6 skeletal muscle
T-173.5 skin
T-171.6 soft tissue
T-171.6 subcutaneous tissue

- C -

M-8510/3 C cell carcinoma (T-193.9)

T-153.4 Caecum

Calcifying
M-9340/0 epithelial odontogenic tumor (T-170._)
M-8110/0 epithelioma of Malherbe (T-173._)
M-9301/0 odontogenic cyst (T-170._)

M------- Calcinosis, tumoral (*SNOMED M-55520*)

Calf
T-195.5 NOS
T-173.7 NOS (carcinoma, melanoma, nevus)
T-171.3 NOS (sarcoma, lipoma)
T-171.3 adipose tissue
T-171.3 connective tissue
T-171.3 fatty tissue
T-171.3 fibrous tissue
T-171.3 muscle
T-171.3 skeletal muscle
T-173.7 skin
T-171.3 soft tissue
T-171.3 subcutaneous tissue
T-171.3 tendon
T-171.3 tendon sheath

T-170.0 Calvarium
T-189.1 Calyces, renal
T-189.1 Calyx, renal

Canal
T-154.2 anal
T-173.2 auditory, NOS
T-173.2 auditory, external
T-173.2 auricular, NOS
T-173.2 auricular, external
T-180.0 cervical
T-173.2 ear
T-180.0 endocervical
T-151.1 pyloric

T-155.1 Canaliculus, biliary

M-8000/3 Cancer (*see Introduction page xv*)

Canthus
T-173.1 NOS
T-173.1 inner
T-173.1 outer

M-9131/0 Capillary hemangioma
M-9171/0 Capillary lymphangioma

T-191.0 Capsule, internal

Carcinoid

M-8240/1	NOS
M-8244/3	composite
M-8243/3	goblet cell
M-8240/3	malignant
M-9091/1	strumal (T-183.0)
M-8240/1	tumor, NOS
M-8241/1	tumor, argentaffin, NOS
M-8241/3	tumor, argentaffin, malignant
M-8240/3	tumor, malignant
M-8242/1	tumor, non-argentaffin, NOS
M-8242/3	tumor, non-argentaffin, malignant

M-9091/1 Carcinoid and struma ovarii (T-183.0)

M-8240/3 Carcinoid type bronchial adenoma (T-162._)

Carcinoma (see also Adenocarcinoma)

M-8010/3	NOS
M-8010/6	NOS, metastatic
M-8280/3	acidophil (T-194.3)
M-8281/3	acidophil-basophil, mixed (T-194.3)
M-8550/3	acinar
M-8550/3	acinar cell
M-8200/3	adenocystic
M-8200/3	adenoid cystic
M-8075/3	adenoid squamous cell
M-8560/3	adenosquamous
M-8390/3	adnexal (T-173._)
M-8370/3	adrenal cortical (T-194.0)
M-8251/3	alveolar
M-8250/3	alveolar cell (T-162._)
M-8021/3	anaplastic type, NOS
M-8090/3	basal cell, NOS (T-173._)
M-8093/3	basal cell, fibroepithelial type (T-173._)
M-8092/3	basal cell, morphea type (T-173._)
M-8090/3	basal cell, pigmented
M-8091/3	basal cell, multicentric (T-173._)
M-8094/3	basal-squamous cell, mixed (T-173._)
M-8123/3	basaloid
M-8300/3	basophil (T-194.3)
M-8281/3	basophil-acidophil, mixed (T-194.3)
M-8094/3	basosquamous (T-173._)
M-8160/3	bile duct (T-155._)
M-8180/3	bile duct and hepatocellular, mixed (T-155.0)
M-8081/2	Bowen's type, intraepidermal squamous cell
M-8250/3	bronchiolar (T-162._)
M-8250/3	bronchiolo-alveolar (T-162._)
M-8510/3	C cell (T-193.9)
M-8420/3	ceruminous (T-173.2)
M-8270/3	chromophobe (T-194.3)
M-8310/3	clear cell
M-8124/3	cloacogenic
M-8480/3	colloid

Carcinoma (Cont'd)

M-8201/3	cribriform
M-8145/3	diffuse type (T-151._)
M-8500/3	duct, NOS
M-8500/3	duct, infiltrating (T-174._)
M-8541/3	duct, infiltrating and Paget's disease (T-174._)
M-8500/3	duct cell
M-8500/3	ductal
M-8521/3	ductular, infiltrating
M-9070/3	embryonal, NOS
M-9101/3	embryonal, combined with choriocarcinoma
M-9071/3	embryonal, infantile type
M-9072/3	embryonal, polyembryonal type
M-9081/3	embryonal and teratoma, mixed
M-8380/3	endometrioid
M-8280/3	eosinophil (T-194.3)
M-8070/3	epidermoid, NOS
M-8071/3	epidermoid, keratinizing type
M-8072/3	epidermoid, large cell, non-keratinizing type
M-8052/3	epidermoid, papillary
M-8073/3	epidermoid, small cell, non-keratinizing type
M-8074/3	epidermoid, spindle cell type
M-8051/3	epidermoid, verrucous
M-8560/3	epidermoid and adenocarcinoma, mixed
M-8330/3	follicular, NOS (T-193.9)
M-8340/3	follicular and papillary (T-193.9)
M-8340/3	follicular and papillary, mixed (T-193.9)
M-8332/3	follicular, moderately differentiated type (T-193.9)
M-8331/3	follicular, pure follicle type (T-193.9)
M-8332/3	follicular, trabecular type (T-193.9)
M-8331/3	follicular, well differentiated type (T-193.9)
M-8480/3	gelatinous
M-8031/3	giant cell
M-8030/3	giant cell and spindle cell
M-8320/3	granular cell
M-8620/3	granulosa cell (T-183.0)
M-8170/3	hepatocellular, NOS (T-155.0)
M-8180/3	hepatocellular and bile duct, mixed (T-155.0)
M-8180/3	hepatocellular and cholangiocarcinoma, combined (T-155.0)
M-8290/3	Hürthle cell (T-193.9)
M-8210/3	in adenomatous polyp
M-8940/3	in pleomorphic adenoma
M-8010/2	in-situ, NOS
M-8070/2	in-situ, epidermoid, NOS
M-8076/2	in-situ, epidermoid with questionable stromal invasion (T-180._)
M-8500/2	in-situ, intraduct
M-8520/2	in-situ, lobular (T-174._)
M-8050/2	in-situ, papillary

Carcinoma (Cont'd)

M-8070/2	in-situ, squamous cell, NOS
M-8076/2	in-situ, squamous cell with questionable stromal invasion (T-180._)
M-8120/2	in-situ, transitional cell
M-9071/3	infantile type, embryonal
M-8500/3	infiltrating duct (T-174._)
M-8541/3	infiltrating duct and Paget's disease (T-174._)
M-8521/3	infiltrating ductular
M-8520/3	infiltrating lobular (T-174._)
M-8530/3	inflammatory (T-174._)
M-8144/3	intestinal type (T-151._)
M-8504/2	intracystic, non-infiltrating
M-8500/2	intraductal, NOS
M-8500/2	intraductal, non-infiltrating, NOS
M-8503/2	intraductal, non-infiltrating, papillary
M-8070/2	intraepidermal, NOS
M-8081/2	intraepidermal, squamous cell, Bowen's type (T-173._)
M-8010/2	intraepithelial, NOS
M-8070/2	intraepithelial, squamous cell
M-9270/3	intraosseous (T-170.1)
M-8150/3	islet cell (T-157._)
M-8502/3	juvenile, breast (T-174._)
M-8012/3	large cell, NOS
M-8072/3	large cell, squamous cell, non-keratinizing
M-8170/3	liver cell (T-155.0)
M-8520/3	lobular, NOS (T-174._)
M-8520/3	lobular, infiltrating (T-174._)
M-8520/2	lobular, non-infiltrating (T-174._)
M-8082/3	lymphoepithelial
M-8510/3	medullary, NOS
M-8511/3	medullary with amyloid stroma (T-193.9)
M-8512/3	medullary with lymphoid stroma (T-174._)
M-9110/3	mesometanephric
M-8010/6	metastatic, NOS
M-8490/6	metastatic, signet ring cell
M-8095/3	metatypical (T-173._)
M-8076/3	micro-invasive squamous cell
M-8481/3	mucin-producing
M-8481/3	mucin-secreting
M-8480/3	mucinous
M-8430/3	mucoepidermoid
M-8480/3	mucoid
M-8480/3	mucous
M-8504/2	non-infiltrating, intracystic
M-8500/2	non-infiltrating, intraductal, NOS
M-8503/2	non-infiltrating, intraductal papillary
M-8520/2	non-infiltrating, lobular (T-174._)
M-8350/3	nonencapsulated sclerosing (T-193.9)

Carcinoma (Cont'd)

M-8042/3	oat cell (T-162._)
M-9270/3	odontogenic (T-170._)
M-8290/3	oncocytic
M-8050/3	papillary, NOS
M-8340/3	papillary and follicular (T-193.9)
M-8340/3	papillary and follicular, mixed (T-193.9)
M-8052/3	papillary, epidermoid
M-8503/2	papillary, intraductal, non-infiltrating
M-8461/3	papillary, serous surface (T-183.0)
M-8052/3	papillary squamous cell
M-8130/3	papillary transitional cell
M-8510/3	parafollicular cell (T-193.9)
M-8022/3	pleomorphic
M-8034/3	polygonal cell
M-8033/3	pseudosarcomatous
M-8075/3	pseudoglandular, squamous cell
M-8312/3	renal cell (T-189.0)
M-8041/3	reserve cell
M-8041/3	round cell
M-8121/3	Schneiderian
M-8141/3	scirrhous
M-8410/3	sebaceous (T-173._)
M-8010/6	secondary
M-8502/3	secretory, breast (T-174._)
M-8461/3	serous surface papillary (T-183.0)
M-8640/3	Sertoli cell (T-186._)
M-8490/3	signet ring cell
M-8490/6	signet ring cell, metastatic
M-8231/3	simplex
M-8390/3	skin appendage (T-173._)
M-8041/3	small cell, NOS
M-8043/3	small cell, fusiform cell type
M-8073/3	small cell, squamous cell, non-keratinizing type
M-8230/3	solid, NOS
M-8511/3	solid with amyloid stroma (T-193.9)
M-8035/3	spheroidal cell
M-8032/3	spindle cell
M-8030/3	spindle cell and giant cell
M-8070/3	spinous cell
M-8070/3	squamous
M-8070/3	squamous cell, NOS
M-8070/6	squamous cell, NOS, metastatic
M-8075/3	squamous cell, adenoid
M-8071/3	squamous cell, keratinizing type, NOS
M-8071/3	squamous cell, large cell, keratinizing type
M-8072/3	squamous cell, large cell, non-keratinizing type
M-8076/3	squamous cell, micro-invasive (T-180._)
M-8072/3	squamous cell, non-keratinizing type, NOS
M-8052/3	squamous cell, papillary

Carcinoma (Cont'd)

M-8075/3	squamous cell, pseudoglandular
M-8073/3	squamous cell, small cell, non-keratinizing type
M-8074/3	squamous cell, spindle cell type
M-8051/3	squamous cell, verrucous
M-8560/3	squamous cell and adenocarcinoma, mixed
M-8400/3	sweat gland (T-173._)
M-8250/3	terminal bronchiolar (T-162._)
M-8600/3	theca cell (T-183.0)
M-8580/3	thymic (T-164.0)
M-8190/3	trabecular
M-8120/3	transitional
M-8120/3	transitional cell, NOS
M-8130/3	transitional cell, papillary
M-8122/3	transitional cell, spindle cell type
M-8211/3	tubular
M-8020/3	undifferentiated type, NOS
M-8120/3	urothelial
M-8051/3	verrucous, NOS
M-8051/3	verrucous, epidermoid
M-8051/3	verrucous, squamous cell
M-8322/3	water-clear cell (T-194.1)
M-8573/3	with apocrine metaplasia
M-8141/3	with productive fibrosis
M-9110/3	Wolffian duct

M-8010/9	Carcinomatosis
M-8980/3	Carcinosarcoma, NOS
M-8981/3	Carcinosarcoma, embryonal type

T-151.0	Cardia, NOS
T-151.0	Cardia, gastric
T-164.1	Cardiac atrium
T-164.1	Cardiac ventricle
T-151.0	Cardio-esophageal junction
T-162.2	Carina
T-171.0	Carotid artery
T-194.5	Carotid body

M-8692/1	Carotid body paraganglioma (T-194.5)
M-8692/1	Carotid body tumor (T-194.5)

T-170.5	Carpal bone

Cartilage

T-170.9	NOS
T-170.9	articular, NOS
T-161.3	arytenoid
T-171.0	auricular
T-170.3	costal
T-161.3	cricoid
T-161.3	cuneiform

Cartilage (Cont'd)

T-171.0	ear
T-161.3	laryngeal
T-160.0	nasal
T-170.7	semilunar
T-161.3	thyroid

M-9210/0	Cartilaginous exostosis (T-170._)

T-192.2	Cauda equina

M-9121/0	Cavernous hemangioma
M-9172/0	Cavernous lymphangioma

Cavity

T-145.9	buccal
T-160.0	nasal *(excludes Nose, NOS T-195.0)*
T-145.9	oral
T-158.9	peritoneal
T-160.1	tympanic

T-153.4	Cecum
T-171.5	Celiac artery
T-196.2	Celiac lymph node

Cellular

M-8790/0	blue nevus (T-173._)
M-9020/0	intracanalicular fibroadenoma (T-174._)
M-8892/1	leiomyoma

M-------	Cemental dysplasia, periapical *(SNOMED M-74870)*
M-9274/0	Cementifying fibroma (T-170._)
M-9273/0	Cementoblastoma, benign (T-170._)
M-9272/0	Cementoma, NOS (T-170._)
M-9275/0	Cementoma, gigantiform (T-170._)
M-------	Central giant cell granuloma *(SNOMED M-44130)*
M-9321/0	Central odontogenic epithelial hamartoma (T-170._)

Central

T-192.9	nervous system
T-174.1	portion of breast
T-191.0	white matter

M-9480/3	Cerebellar sarcoma, NOS (T-191.6)
M-9471/3	Cerebellar sarcoma, arachnoidal, circumscribed (T-191.6)

T-191.6   Cerebellopontine angle
T-191.6   Cerebellum, NOS
T-191.6   Cerebellum, vermis

Cerebral
T-191.0   cortex
T-191.0   hemisphere
T-192.1   meninges
T-191.7   peduncle
T-191.5   ventricle
T-191.0   white matter

T-191.0   Cerebrum
T-173.2   Ceruminal gland

Ceruminous
M-8420/3   adenocarcinoma (T-173.2)
M-8420/0   adenoma (T-173.2)
M-8420/3   carcinoma (T-173.2)

Cervical
T-180.0   canal
T-192.2   cord
T-150.0   esophagus
T-196.0   lymph node
T-171.0   plexus
T-195.0   region, NOS
T-180.8   stump

Cervical region
T-195.0   NOS
T-173.4   NOS (carcinoma, melanoma, nevus)
T-171.0   NOS (sarcoma, lipoma)
T-171.0   adipose tissue
T-171.0   connective tissue
T-171.0   fatty tissue
T-171.0   fibrous tissue
T-173.4   skin
T-171.0   soft tissue
T-171.0   subcutaneous tissue

Cervix
T-180.9   NOS
T-180.8   squamocolumnar junction
T-180.9   uteri
T-180.9   uterine

M-------   Chalazion (SNOMED M-43000)

Cheek
T-195.0   NOS
T-173.3   NOS (carcinoma, melanoma, nevus)
T-171.0   NOS (sarcoma, lipoma)
T-171.0   adipose tissue
T-171.0   connective tissue
T-173.3   external
T-171.0   fatty tissue
T-171.0   fibrous tissue
T-145.0   internal
T-145.0   mucosa
T-173.3   skin
T-171.0   soft tissue
T-171.0   subcutaneous tissue

M-8693/1 Chemodectoma

Chest
T-195.1   NOS
T-173.5   NOS (carcinoma, melanoma, nevus)
T-171.4   NOS (sarcoma, lipoma)
T-171.4   connective tissue
T-171.4   fibrous tissue
T-173.5   skin
T-171.4   soft tissue
T-171.4   subcutaneous tissue

Chest wall
T-195.1   NOS
T-173.5   NOS (carcinoma, melanoma, nevus)
T-171.4   NOS (sarcoma, lipoma)
T-171.4   adipose tissue
T-171.4   connective tissue
T-171.4   fatty tissue
T-171.4   fibrous tissue
T-171.4   muscle
T-171.4   skeletal muscle
T-173.5   skin
T-171.4   soft tissue
T-171.4   subcutaneous tissue

T-192.0   Chiasm, optic

M-8321/0 Chief cell adenoma (T-194.1)

Chin
T-173.3   NOS
T-173.3   NOS (carcinoma, melanoma, nevus)
T-171.0   NOS (sarcoma, lipoma)
T-171.0   connective tissue
T-171.0   fibrous tissue

Chin (Cont'd)
T-173.3   skin
T-171.0   soft tissue
T-171.0   subcutaneous tissue

M-9930/3 Chloroma

T-147.3   Choana

M-8160/3 Cholangiocarcinoma (T-155._)
M-8180/3 Cholangiocarcinoma and hepatocellular
           carcinoma, combined (T-155.0)

T-155.1   Cholangiole

M-8160/0 Cholangioma (T-155._)

T-156.1   Choledochal duct

M------- Cholesteatoma, NOS (SNOMED M-72900)
M------- Cholesteatoma, epidermoid
           (SNOMED M-72900)
M-9181/3 Chondroblastic osteosarcoma (T-170._)
M-9230/0 Chondroblastoma, NOS (T-170._)
M-9230/3 Chondroblastoma, malignant (T-170._)
M-8940/0 Chondroid syringoma

Chondroma
M-9220/0   NOS (T-170._)
M-9221/0   juxtacortical (T-170._)
M-9221/0   periosteal (T-170._)

M-9220/1 Chondromatosis, NOS
M------- Chondromatosis, synovial (SNOMED M-73670)
M-9230/0 Chondromatous giant cell tumor (T-170._)
M-9241/0 Chondromyxoid fibroma (T-170._)

Chondrosarcoma
M-9220/3   NOS (T-170._)
M-9221/3   juxtacortical (T-170._)
M-9240/3   mesenchymal

M-9370/3 Chordoma
M-9100/1 Chorioadenoma (T-181.9)
M-9100/1 Chorioadenoma destruens (T-181.9)
M-9120/0 Chorioangioma (T-181.9)
M-9100/3 Choriocarcinoma
M-9101/3 Choriocarcinoma, combined with embryonal
           carcinoma
M-9101/3 Choriocarcinoma, combined with teratoma
M-9100/3 Chorioepithelioma
M-9100/3 Chorionepithelioma

M------- Choristoma (SNOMED M-75520)

T-190.6   Choroid
T-191.5   Choroid plexus

Choroid plexus papilloma
M-9390/0   NOS (T-191.5)
M-9390/3   anaplastic type (T-191.5)
M-9390/3   malignant (T-191.5)

M-8700/0 Chromaffin paraganglioma
M-8700/0 Chromaffin tumor
M-8700/0 Chromaffinoma

Chromophobe
M-8270/3   adenocarcinoma (T-194.3)
M-8270/0   adenoma (T-194.3)
M-8270/3   carcinoma (T-194.3)

Chronic
M-9842/3   erythremia (T-169._)
M-9970/1   lymphoproliferative disease
M-9960/1   myeloproliferative disease (T-169._)
M-9863/3   myelosis (T-169._)

M------- Cicatricial fibromatosis (SNOMED M-76170)

T-190.0   Ciliary body

M-9471/3 Circumscribed arachnoidal cerebellar sarcoma
           (T-191.6)

T-170.3   Clavicle

Clear cell
M-------   acanthoma (SNOMED M-72530)
M-8310/3   adenocarcinoma, NOS
M-8310/3   adenocarcinoma, mesonephroid type
M-8313/0   adenofibroma
M-8310/0   adenoma
M-8310/3   carcinoma
M-8313/0   cystadenofibroma
M-8402/0   hidradenoma (T-173._)
M-9044/3   sarcoma of tendons and aponeuroses
           (T-171._)
M-8373/0   type, adrenal cortical adenoma (T-194.0)

T-146.8   Cleft, branchial (site of neoplasm)
T-184.3   Clitoris

M-8124/3 Cloacogenic carcinoma

T-154.8	Cloacogenic zone		**Common** (Cont'd)	
T-196.5	Cloquet's lymph node	T-156.1	duct	
T-194.6	Coccygeal body	T-196.2	duct lymph node	
T-194.6	Coccygeal glomus			
T-170.6	Coccyx	M-8371/0	Compact cell type, adrenal cortical adenoma (T-194.0)	

M-9230/0 Codman's tumor (T-170._)

M-9282/0	Complex odontoma (T-170._)
M-8244/3	Composite carcinoid
M-8760/0	Compound nevus (T-173._)
M-9281/0	Compound odontoma (T-170._)

T-196.2 Colic lymph node

M------- Colitis cystica profunda (*SNOMED M-43800*)

T-173.2 Concha

Colloid

M-8480/3	adenocarcinoma
M-8334/0	adenoma (T-193.9)
M-8480/3	carcinoma
M-------	goiter (*SNOMED M-71620*)

Condyloma

M-------	NOS (*SNOMED M-76700*)
M-------	acuminatum (*SNOMED M-76720*)
M-------	giant (*SNOMED M-76730*)

Colon

T-153.9	NOS
T-153.5	appendix
T-153.6	ascending
T-153.4	cecum
T-153.2	descending
T-153.0	hepatic flexure
T-153.2	left
T-153.3	pelvic
T-154.0	rectosigmoid
T-153.6	right
T-153.3	sigmoid
T-153.3	sigmoid flexure
T-153.7	splenic flexure
T-153.1	transverse

Congenital

M-------	cyst, NOS (*SNOMED M-26500*)
M-------	dysplasia, NOS (*SNOMED M-20020*)
M-8814/3	fibrosarcoma
M-------	melanosis (*SNOMED M-25110*)

T-190.3 Conjunctiva

T-154.0	Colon and rectum
T-170.2	Column, spinal
T-170.2	Column, vertebral (*excludes Sacrum and Coccyx T-170.6*)
T-173.3	Columnella

Connective tissue

T-171.9	NOS
T-171.5	abdomen
T-171.5	abdominal wall
T-171.3	ankle
T-171.2	antecubital space
T-171.2	arm
T-171.4	axilla
T-171.7	back
T-171.6	buttock
T-171.3	calf
T-171.0	cervical region
T-171.0	cheek
T-171.4	chest
T-171.4	chest wall
T-171.0	chin
T-171.2	elbow
T-171.0	face
T-171.2	finger
T-171.7	flank
T-171.3	foot
T-171.2	forearm
T-171.0	forehead
T-171.6	gluteal region

M-8180/3 Combined hepatocellular carcinoma and cholangiocarcinoma (T-155.0)

M-8501/3 Comedocarcinoma, NOS (T-174._)

M-8501/2 Comedocarcinoma, non-infiltrating (T-174._)

Commissure

T-140.6	labial
T-161.0	laryngeal
T-140.6	lip

Common

T-156.1	bile duct

Connective tissue (Cont'd)

T-171.6	groin
T-171.2	hand
T-171.0	head
T-171.3	heel
T-171.3	hip
T-171.4	infraclavicular region
T-171.6	inguinal region
T-171.3	knee
T-171.3	leg
T-171.0	neck
T-190.1	orbit
T-171.6	pelvis
T-171.6	perineum
T-171.3	popliteal space
T-171.0	pterygoid fossa
T-171.6	sacrococcygeal region
T-171.0	scalp
T-171.4	scapular region
T-171.2	shoulder
T-171.0	supraclavicular region
T-171.0	temple
T-171.3	thigh
T-171.4	thoracic wall
T-171.4	thorax (*excludes Thymus, Heart and Mediastinum T-164.__*)
T-171.2	thumb
T-171.3	toe
T-171.7	trunk
T-171.5	umbilicus
T-171.2	wrist

T-192.2	Conus medullaris
T-171.2	Coracobrachialis muscle

Cord

T-192.2	cervical
T-161.1	false
T-192.2	lumbar
T-192.2	sacral
T-187.6	spermatic
T-192.2	spinal
T-192.2	thoracic
T-161.0	true

Cord, vocal

T-161.0	NOS
T-161.1	false
T-161.0	true

T-190.4	Cornea, NOS
T-190.4	Cornea, limbus

Corpus

T-191.8	callosum
T-187.3	cavernosum
T-151.4	gastric
T-187.3	penis
T-151.4	stomach
T-191.0	striatum
T-182.0	uteri

T-194.0	Cortex, adrenal
T-191.0	Cortex, cerebral
T-170.3	Costal cartilage
T-170.3	Costovertebral joint
T-189.3	Cowper's gland

Cranial

T-170.0	bone
T-192.1	dura mater
T-192.1	meninges
T-192.0	nerve
T-192.1	pia mater

Cranial fossa

T-191.9	NOS
T-191.9	anterior
T-191.9	middle
T-191.9	posterior

T-194.3	Craniopharyngeal duct
M-9350/1	Craniopharyngioma (T-194.3)
M-8201/3	Cribriform carcinoma
T-148.0	Cricoid, NOS
T-161.3	Cricoid cartilage
T-148.0	Cricopharynx
T-190.0	Crystalline lens
T-196.3	Cubital lymph node
T-158.8	Cul de sac
T-161.3	Cuneiform cartilage
M-------	Cutaneous horn (*SNOMED M-72840*)
M-8200/3	Cylindroid type adenocarcinoma
M-8200/3	Cylindroid type bronchial adenoma (T-162.__)

Cylindroma

M-8200/3	NOS (*except Cylindroma of Skin M-8200/0*)
M-8200/0	eccrine dermal (**T-173.__**)
M-8200/0	skin (**T-173.__**)

Cyst

M-------	NOS *(SNOMED M-33400)*
M-------	aneurysmal bone *(SNOMED M-33640)*
M-------	congenital, NOS *(SNOMED M-26500)*
M-------	dentigerous *(SNOMED M-26560)*
M-9084/0	dermoid
M-9084/3	dermoid with malignant transformation (T-183.0)
M-------	enterogenous *(SNOMED M-26660)*
M-------	epidermoid *(SNOMED M-33410)*
M-------	eruption *(SNOMED M-26550)*
M-------	follicular, jaw *(SNOMED M-26560)*
M-------	ganglion *(SNOMED M-33600)*
M-------	gingival, NOS *(SNOMED M-26540)*
M-------	gingival, odontogenic *(SNOMED M-26540)*
M-------	nasopalatine duct *(SNOMED M-26600)*
M-------	pilar *(SNOMED M-33470)*
M-------	primordial *(SNOMED M-26530)*
M-------	radicular *(SNOMED M-43800)*
M-------	sebaceous *(SNOMED M-33430)*
M-------	solitary *(SNOMED M-33404)*
M-------	thyroglossal duct *(SNOMED M-26500)*

Cyst, odontogenic

M-------	NOS *(SNOMED M-26520)*
M-9301/0	calcifying (T-170._)
M-------	dentigerous *(SNOMED M-26560)*
M-------	eruptive *(SNOMED M-26550)*
M-------	gingival *(SNOMED M-26540)*
M-------	primordial *(SNOMED M-26530)*

Cystadenocarcinoma

M-8440/3	NOS
M-8161/3	bile duct (T-155._)
M-8380/3	endometrioid
M-8470/3	mucinous, NOS (T-183.0)
M-8450/3	papillary, NOS (T-183.0)
M-8471/3	papillary mucinous (T-183.0)
M-8471/3	papillary pseudomucinous (T-183.0)
M-8460/3	papillary serous (T-183.0)
M-8470/3	pseudomucinous, NOS (T-183.0)
M-8441/3	serous, NOS (T-183.0)

Cystadenofibroma

M-9013/0	NOS (T-183.0)
M-8313/0	clear cell
M-8381/0	endometrioid, NOS (T-183.0)
M-8381/1	endometrioid, borderline malignancy (T-183.0)
M-8381/3	endometrioid, malignant (T-183.0)
M-9015/0	mucinous (T-183.0)
M-9014/0	serous (T-183.0)

Cystadenoma

M-8440/0	NOS
M-8161/0	bile duct (T-155._)
M-8380/0	endometrioid, NOS
M-8380/1	endometrioid, borderline malignancy
M-8561/0	lymphomatosum, papillary (T-142._)
M-8470/0	mucinous, NOS (T-183.0)
M-8470/1	mucinous, borderline malignancy (T-183.0)
M-8450/0	papillary, NOS (T-183.0)
M-8450/1	papillary, borderline malignancy (T-183.0)
M-8471/0	papillary mucinous, NOS (T-183.0)
M-8471/1	papillary mucinous, borderline malignancy (T-183.0)
M-8471/0	papillary pseudomucinous, NOS (T-183.0)
M-8471/1	papillary pseudomucinous, borderline malignancy (T-183.0)
M-8460/0	papillary serous, NOS (T-183.0)
M-8460/1	papillary serous, borderline malignancy (T-183.0)
M-8470/0	pseudomucinous, NOS (T-183.0)
M-8470/1	pseudomucinous, borderline malignancy (T-183.0)
M-8441/0	serous, NOS (T-183.0)
M-8441/1	serous, borderline malignancy (T-183.0)

Cystic

M-9400/3	astrocytoma (T-191._)
M-------	disease of the breast *(SNOMED M-74320)*
M-9173/0	hygroma
M-9173/0	lymphangioma
M-9080/0	teratoma, NOS
M-9080/0	teratoma, adult
T-156.1	Cystic bile duct
T-156.1	Cystic duct
M-------	Cystitis cystica *(SNOMED M-73370)*
M-------	Cystitis, papillary *(SNOMED M-76820)*

Cystoma

M-8440/0	NOS
M-8470/0	mucinous (T-183.0)
M-8441/0	serous (T-183.0)

Cystosarcoma phyllodes

M-9020/1	NOS (T-174._)
M-9020/0	benign (T-174._)
M-9020/3	malignant (T-174._)

- D -

M------- Decidual change *(SNOMED M-79500)*

T-171.2 Deltoideus muscle

M------- Dentigerous cyst *(SNOMED M-26560)*
M-9271/0 Dentinoma (T-170._)
M-8760/0 Dermal and epidermal nevus (T-173._)
M-8200/0 Dermal eccrine cylindroma (T-173._)
M-8750/0 Dermal nevus (T-173._)

Dermatofibroma
M-8832/0 NOS (T-173._)
M-8832/0 lenticulare (T-173._)
M-8832/1 protuberans (T-173._)

M-8832/3 Dermatofibrosarcoma, NOS (T-173._)
M-8832/3 Dermatofibrosarcoma protuberans (T-173._)

Dermoid
M-9084/0 NOS
M-9084/0 cyst
M-9084/3 cyst with malignant transformation (T-183.0)

T-186.9 Descended testis
T-153.2 Descending colon

Desmoid
M-8821/1 NOS
M-8822/1 abdominal
M-8821/1 extra-abdominal

M-8823/1 Desmoplastic fibroma
M-9471/3 Desmoplastic medulloblastoma (T-191.6)
M-9841/3 Di Guglielmo's disease (T-169._)

T-171.4 Diaphragm
T-196.1 Diaphragmatic lymph node

M-___/_(1) Differentiated *(see Grading code, page 20)*

Differentiated type
M-8851/3 liposarcoma
M-9511/3 retinoblastoma (T-190.5)
M-9080/0 teratoma

Diffuse
M-9632/3 germinoblastic sarcoma
M-9614/3 germinoblastoma
M-8505/0 intraductal papillomatosis
M------- lipomatosis *(SNOMED M-74103)*
M-9630/3 lymphoblastic lymphoma
M-9630/3 lymphoblastoma
M-9620/3 lymphocytic lymphoma, NOS
M-9630/3 lymphocytic lymphoma, poorly differentiated
M-9610/3 lymphosarcoma, NOS
M-9630/3 lymphosarcoma, lymphoblastic
M-9620/3 lymphosarcoma, lymphocytic, NOS
M-9621/3 lymphosarcoma, lymphocytic, intermediate differentiation
M-9611/3 lymphosarcoma, lymphoplasmacytic
M-9613/3 lymphosarcoma, mixed cell type
M-9611/3 lymphosarcoma with plasmacytoid differentiation
M-9590/3 malignant lymphoma, NOS *(see also Malignant lymphoma, diffuse)*
M-9530/1 meningiomatosis (T-192._)
M-9613/3 reticulolymphosarcoma
M-8145/3 type, adenocarcinoma (T-151._)
M-8145/3 type, carcinoma (T-151._)

T-159.9 Digestive organs, NOS

M-9501/3 Diktyoma

T-170.2 Disc, intervertebral
T-150.5 Distal third of esophagus
T-152.3 Diverticulum, Meckel's *(site of neoplasm)*
T-188.1 Dome, urinary bladder

Dorsal surface
T-141.1 anterior tongue
T-141.1 tongue, NOS
T-141.1 tongue, anterior 2/3
T-141.0 tongue, base

T-158.8 Douglas's pouch

Duct

M-8500/3	adenocarcinoma, NOS
M-8500/3	adenocarcinoma, infiltrating (T-174._)
M-8503/0	adenoma, NOS
M-8500/3	carcinoma, NOS
M-8500/3	carcinoma, infiltrating (T-174._)
M-8541/3	carcinoma, infiltrating and Paget's disease (T-174._)
M-8500/3	cell carcinoma
M-------	ectasia, mammary (SNOMED M-32100)
M-8506/0	papillomatosis, subareolar (T-174.0)
M-9110/0	Wolffian, adenoma
M-9110/3	Wolffian, carcinoma

Duct

T-156.1	bile, NOS
T-156.1	biliary, NOS
T-156.1	choledochal
T-156.1	common
T-156.1	common bile
T-194.3	craniopharyngeal
T-156.1	cystic
T-156.1	cystic bile
T-156.1	extrahepatic bile
T-184.0	Gartner's
T-156.1	hepatic
T-156.1	hepatic bile
T-155.1	intrahepatic bile
T-190.7	lacrimal, NOS
T-190.7	nasal lacrimal
T-190.7	nasolacrimal
T-157.3	pancreatic
T-142.0	parotid gland
T-157.3	Santorini's
T-142.0	Stensen's
T-142.2	sublingual gland
T-142.1	submaxillary gland
T-171.4	thoracic
T-193.9	thyroglossal
T-142.1	Wharton's
T-157.3	Wirsung's

M-8500/3	Ductal carcinoma
M-8503/0	Ductal papilloma
M-8521/3	Ductular carcinoma, infiltrating

T-152.0	Duodenum

Dura mater

T-192.1	NOS
T-192.1	cranial
T-192.3	spinal

T-192.1	Dura, NOS

M-------	Dysgenesis, NOS (SNOMED M-20000)
M-9060/3	Dysgerminoma
M-8052/0	Dyskeratotic papilloma

Dysplasia

M-------	NOS (SNOMED M-74000)
M-------	congenital, NOS (SNOMED M-20020)
M-------	fibrous, NOS (SNOMED M-74910)
M-------	mild (SNOMED M-74006)
M-------	moderate (SNOMED M-74007)
M-------	periapical cemental (SNOMED M-74870)
M-------	severe (SNOMED M-74008)

- E -

Ear

T-173.2	NOS
T-173.2	canal
T-171.0	cartilage
T-173.2	external
T-160.1	inner
T-173.2	lobule
T-160.1	middle
T-173.2	skin

T-173.2	Earlobe

M-9210/0	Ecchondroma (T-170._)
M-9210/1	Ecchondrosis (T-170._)

Eccrine

M-8402/0	acrospiroma (T-173._)
M-8200/0	dermal cylindroma (T-173._)
M-8402/0	poroma (T-173._)
M-8403/0	spiradenoma (T-173._)

M-------	Ectasia, mammary duct (SNOMED M-32100)
M-------	Ectopia, NOS (SNOMED M-26000)
M-------	Ectopic glial tissue (SNOMED M-26160)
T-186.0	Ectopic testis (site of neoplasm)
M-8820/0	Elastofibroma

Elbow

T-195.4	NOS
T-173.6	NOS (carcinoma, melanoma, nevus)
T-171.2	NOS (sarcoma, lipoma)
T-171.2	connective tissue
T-171.2	fibrous tissue
T-170.4	joint
T-173.6	skin
T-171.2	soft tissue
T-171.2	subcutaneous tissue

Embryonal

M-9070/3	adenocarcinoma
M-8191/0	adenoma
M-9070/3	carcinoma, NOS
M-9101/3	carcinoma, combined with choriocarcinoma
M-9071/3	carcinoma, infantile type
M-9072/3	carcinoma, polyembryonal type
M-9081/3	carcinoma and teratoma, mixed
M-8970/3	hepatoma (T-155.0)
M-8852/3	liposarcoma
M-------	rest, NOS (SNOMED M-26300)
M-8910/3	rhabdomyosarcoma
M-8991/3	sarcoma
M-9080/3	teratoma
M-8981/3	type carcinosarcoma

M-9220/0 Enchondroma (T-170._)
M------- Endemic goiter (SNOMED M-71660)

T-164.1 Endocardium
T-180.0 Endocervical canal
T-180.0 Endocervical gland
T-180.0 Endocervix

M-8360/1 Endocrine adenomas, multiple
M-8360/1 Endocrine adenomatosis

T-194.9 Endocrine gland, NOS
T-194.8 Endocrine glands, multiple

M-9071/3 Endodermal sinus tumor
M-8931/1 Endolymphatic stromal myosis (T-182.0)

T-182.0 Endometrial gland

Endometrial

M-8930/3	sarcoma, NOS (T-182.0)
M-8930/3	stromal sarcoma (T-182.0)
M-8931/1	stromatosis (T-182.0)

T-182.0 Endometrial stroma

Endometrioid

M-8380/3	adenocarcinoma
M-8381/0	adenofibroma, NOS (T-183.0)
M-8381/1	adenofibroma, borderline malignancy (T-183.0)
M-8381/3	adenofibroma, malignant (T-183.0)
M-8380/0	adenoma, NOS
M-8380/1	adenoma, borderline malignancy
M-8380/3	carcinoma
M-8380/3	cystadenocarcinoma
M-8381/0	cystadenofibroma, NOS (T-183.0)
M-8381/1	cystadenofibroma, borderline malignancy (T-183.0)
M-8381/3	cystadenofibroma, malignant (T-183.0)
M-8380/0	cystadenoma, NOS
M-8380/1	cystadenoma, borderline malignancy

M------- Endometrioma (SNOMED M-76540)

Endometriosis

M-------	NOS (SNOMED M-76500)
M-------	external (SNOMED M-76500)
M-------	internal (SNOMED M-76510)
M-8931/1	stromal (T-182.0) ·

T-182.0 Endometrium

M-9111/1 Endosalpingioma
M-9260/3 Endothelial sarcoma of bone (T-170._)
M-9531/0 Endotheliomatous meningioma (T-192._)
M------- Enterogenous cyst (SNOMED M-26660)

Eosinophil

M-8280/3	adenocarcinoma (T-194.3)
M-8280/0	adenoma (T-194.3)
M-8280/3	carcinoma (T-194.3)

M------- Eosinophilic granuloma, NOS (SNOMED M-44050)
M------- Eosinophilic granuloma of bone (SNOMED M-77860)

T-191.5 Ependyma

M-9392/3 Ependymoblastoma (T-191._)

Ependymoma

M-9391/3	NOS (T-191._)
M-9392/3	anaplastic type (T-191._)
M-9391/3	epithelial (T-191._)
M-9394/1	myxopapillary (T-191._)
M-9393/1	papillary (T-191._)

M------- Ephelis *(SNOMED M-57260)*

T-164.1 Epicardium

M-8760/0 Epidermal and dermal nevus (T-173._)

Epidermoid carcinoma
M-8070/3 NOS
M-8560/3 and adenocarcinoma, mixed
M-8070/2 in-situ, NOS
M-8076/2 in-situ with questionable stromal invasion
          (T-180._)
M-8071/3 keratinizing type
M-8072/3 large cell, non-keratinizing type
M-8052/3 papillary
M-8073/3 small cell, non-keratinizing type
M-8074/3 spindle cell type
M-8051/3 verrucous

M------- Epidermoid cholesteatoma
          (SNOMED M-72900)
M------- Epidermoid cyst *(SNOMED M-33410)*

T-187.5 Epididymis
T-192.9 Epidural

Epiglottis
T-161.1 NOS *(excludes Anterior surface of
          epiglottis T-146.4)*
T-146.4 anterior surface
T-161.1 posterior surface

M-9391/1 Epithelial ependymoma (T-191._)
M-8961/3 Epithelial nephroblastoma (T-189.0)

Epithelial tumor
M-8010/0 benign
M-8010/3 malignant
M-9340/0 odontogenic, calcifying (T-170._)

Epithelioid
M-8775/3 and spindle cell melanoma, mixed
M-8770/0 and spindle cell nevus (T-173._)
M-8771/3 cell melanoma
M-8771/3 cell melanosarcoma
M-8770/0 cell nevus (T-173._)
M-8804/3 cell sarcoma
M-9042/3 cell type synovial sarcoma
M-8891/1 leiomyoma
M-8891/3 leiomyosarcoma

Epithelioid mesothelioma
M-9052/3 NOS
M-9052/0 benign
M-9052/3 malignant

Epithelioma
M-8011/3 NOS
M-8100/0 adenoides cysticum (T-173._)
M-8090/3 basal cell (T-173._)
M-8011/0 benign
M-8110/0 calcifying, Malherbe (T-173._)
M-8096/0 intraepidermal, Jadassohn (T-173._)
M-8011/3 malignant
M-8070/3 squamous cell

T-196.3 Epitrochlear lymph node

M-8506/0 Erosive adenomatosis, nipple (T-174.0)
M------- Eruption cyst *(SNOMED M-26550)*
M-9841/3 Erythremia, acute (T-169._)
M-9842/3 Erythremia, chronic (T-169._)
M-9840/3 Erythremic myelosis, NOS (T-169._)
M-9841/3 Erythremic myelosis, acute (T-169._)
M-9840/3 Erythroleukemia (T-169._)
M-8080/2 Erythroplasia, Queyrat's (T-187._)

T-196.1 Esophageal lymph node
T-151.0 Esophagogastric junction

Esophagus
T-150.9 NOS
T-150.2 abdominal
T-150.0 cervical
T-150.5 distal third
T-150.5 lower third
T-150.4 middle third
T-150.3 proximal third
T-150.1 thoracic
T-150.3 upper third

M-9522/3 Esthesioneuroblastoma (T-160._)
M-9521/3 Esthesioneurocytoma (T-160._)
M-9523/3 Esthesioneuroepithelioma (T-160._)

T-170.0 Ethmoid bone
T-160.3 Ethmoid sinus
T-160.1 Eustachian tube

M-9260/3 Ewing's sarcoma (T-170._)
M-9260/3 Ewing's tumor (T-170._)

T-180.1 Exocervix

M-8154/3 Exocrine and islet cell adenocarcinoma, mixed
(T-157._)
M------- Exostosis, NOS (SNOMED M-71440)
M-9210/0 Exostosis, cartilaginous (T-170._)
M-9210/0 Exostosis, osteocartilaginous (T-170._)

External
T-173.2   auditory canal
T-173.2   auditory meatus
T-173.2   auricular canal
T-173.3   cheek
T-173.2   ear
T-184.4   female genitalia
T-173.3   nose
T-180.1   os

External lip
T-140.9   NOS
T-140.1   lower
T-140.0   upper

M------- External endometriosis (SNOMED M-76500)
M-8821/1 Extra-abdominal desmoid
M-8693/1 Extra-adrenal paraganglioma, NOS
M-8693/3 Extra-adrenal paraganglioma, malignant

T-192.9   Extradural
T-190.1   Extra-ocular muscle
T-156.1   Extrahepatic bile duct

M-8542/3 Extramammary Paget's disease (except
Paget's disease of bone)

T-161.1   Extrinsic larynx

Eye
T-190.9   NOS
T-173.1   canthus, NOS
T-173.1   canthus, inner
T-173.1   canthus, outer
T-190.6   choroid
T-190.0   ciliary body
T-190.3   conjunctiva
T-190.1   connective tissue, orbit
T-190.4   cornea, NOS
T-190.4   cornea, limbus
T-190.0   crystalline lens
T-190.1   extra-ocular muscle
T-190.0   eyeball
T-173.3   eyebrow
T-173.1   eyelid
T-190.0   intraocular

Eye (Cont'd)
T-190.0   iris
T-190.2   lacrimal gland
T-190.7   lacrimal duct, NOS
T-190.7   lacrimal duct, nasal
T-190.7   lacrimal sac
T-190.0   lens, crystalline
T-173.1   lid, NOS
T-173.1   lid, lower
T-173.1   lid, upper
T-173.1   Meibomian gland
T-190.1   muscle, extra-ocular
T-190.7   nasal lacrimal duct
T-190.7   nasolacrimal duct
T-192.0   optic nerve
T-190.1   orbit, NOS
T-190.1   orbit, connective tissue
T-190.1   orbit, soft tissue
T-173.1   palpebra
T-190.5   retina
T-190.1   retrobulbar tissue
T-190.0   sclera
T-190.0   uveal tract

T-190.0   Eyeball

- F -

Face
T-195.0   NOS
T-173.3   NOS (carcinoma, melanoma, nevus)
T-171.0   NOS (sarcoma, lipoma)
T-171.0   adipose tissue
T-170.0   bone
T-171.0   connective tissue
T-171.0   fatty tissue
T-171.0   fibrous tissue
T-196.0   lymph node
T-171.0   muscle
T-171.0   skeletal muscle
T-173.3   skin
T-171.0   soft tissue
T-171.0   subcutaneous tissue

Facial
T-170.0   bone
T-196.0   lymph node
T-192.0   nerve

T-183.2   Fallopian tube
T-161.1   False cord
T-161.1   False vocal cord

Falx

T-192.1	NOS
T-192.1	cerebelli
T-192.1	cerebri

M-8220/0	Familial polyposis coli (T-153._)

Fascia

T-171.9	NOS
T-171.2	palmar
T-171.3	plantar

M-8813/0	Fascial fibroma
M-8813/3	Fascial fibrosarcoma

Fasciitis

M-------	infiltrative *(SNOMED M-76130)*
M-------	nodular *(SNOMED M-76130)*
M-------	pseudosarcomatous *(SNOMED M-76130)*
M-------	Fat necrosis *(SNOMED M-54110)*

Fatty tissue

T-171.9	NOS
T-171.5	abdominal wall
T-171.2	antecubital space
T-171.2	arm
T-171.4	axilla
T-171.7	back
T-171.6	buttock
T-171.3	calf
T-171.0	cervical region
T-171.0	cheek
T-171.4	chest wall
T-171.0	face
T-171.7	flank
T-171.3	foot
T-171.2	forearm
T-171.6	gluteal region
T-171.6	groin
T-171.2	hand
T-171.0	head
T-171.3	hip
T-171.4	infraclavicular region
T-171.6	inguinal region
T-171.3	knee
T-171.3	leg
T-171.0	neck
T-171.3	popliteal space
T-171.6	sacrococcygeal region
T-171.0	scalp

Fatty tissue (Cont'd)

T-171.2	shoulder
T-171.0	supraclavicular region
T-171.0	temple
T-171.3	thigh
T-171.7	trunk

T-146.9	Fauces, NOS
T-146.2	Faucial pillar
T-146.0	Faucial tonsil

Female

T-184.9	genital organs, NOS
T-184.9	genital tract, NOS
T-184.4	genitalia, external
T-184.9	genitourinary tract, NOS

Female breast

T-174.9	NOS *(excludes Skin of breast T-173.5)*
T-174.0	areola
T-174.6	axillary tail
T-174.1	central portion
T-174.8	inner
T-174.8	lower
T-174.3	lower-inner quadrant
T-174.5	lower-outer quadrant
T-174.8	midline
T-174.0	nipple
T-174.8	outer
T-174.3	quadrant, lower-inner
T-174.5	quadrant, lower-outer
T-174.2	quadrant, upper-inner
T-174.4	quadrant, upper-outer
T-173.5	skin
T-174.6	tail
T-174.8	upper
T-174.2	upper-inner quadrant
T-174.4	upper-outer quadrant

Femoral

T-171.3	artery
T-196.5	lymph node
T-171.3	nerve

T-170.7	Femur

Fetal

M-8333/0	adenoma (T-193.9)
M-8880/0	fat cell lipoma
M-8881/0	lipoma, NOS
M-8881/0	lipomatosis
M-8903/0	rhabdomyoma

T-181.9   Fetal membranes

M-9420/3 Fibrillary astrocytoma (T-191.__)

Fibroadenoma

M-9010/0   NOS (T-174.__)
M-9020/0   giant, NOS (T-174.__)
M-9011/0   intracanalicular, NOS (T-174.__)
M-9020/0   intracanalicular, cellular (T-174.__)
M-9020/0   intracanalicular, giant (T-174.__)
M-9030/0   juvenile (T-174.__)
M-9012/0   pericanalicular (T-174.__)
M-9020/0   phyllodes (T-174.__)

M-9290/0 Fibroameloblastic odontoma (T-170.__)
M-9532/0 Fibroblastic meningioma (T-192.__)
M-9182/3 Fibroblastic osteosarcoma (T-170.__)
M-9220/3 Fibrochondrosarcoma (T-170.__)
M------- Fibrocystic disease, NOS *(SNOMED M-74320)*

Fibroepithelial

M-------   papilloma *(SNOMED M-76810)*
M-------   polyp *(SNOMED M-76810)*
M-8093/3   type, basal cell carcinoma (T-173.__)

M-8890/0 Fibroid uterus (T-179.9)
M-8851/0 Fibrolipoma
M-8850/3 Fibroliposarcoma

Fibroma

M-8810/0   NOS
M-9330/0   ameloblastic (T-170.__)
M-9274/0   cementifying (T-170.__)
M-9241/0   chondromyxoid (T-170.__)
M-8823/1   desmoplastic
M-8810/0   durum
M-8813/0   fascial
M-8821/1   invasive
M-------   juvenile aponeurotic *(SNOMED M-76150)*
M-8851/0   molle
M-8811/0   myxoid
M-------   non-ossifying *(SNOMED M-74940)*
M-9321/0   odontogenic, NOS (T-170.__)
M-------   odontogenic, peripheral *(SNOMED M-76850)*
M-9262/0   ossifying (T-170.__)
M-8812/0   periosteal (T-170.__)
M-8851/0   soft

Fibromatosis

M-------   NOS *(SNOMED M-76100)*
M-8822/1   abdominal
M-8821/1   aggressive
M-------   cicatricial *(SNOMED M-76170)*
M-------   musculo-aponeurotic *(SNOMED M-76150)*
M-------   pseudosarcomatous *(SNOMED M-76130)*

M-8890/0 Fibromyoma
M-8852/0 Fibromyxolipoma
M-8811/0 Fibromyxoma
M-8811/3 Fibromyxosarcoma
M-9290/0 Fibro-odontoma, ameloblastic (T-170.__)
M-9262/0 Fibro-osteoma (T-170.__)

Fibrosarcoma

M-8810/3   NOS
M-9330/3   ameloblastic (T-170.__)
M-8814/3   congenital
M-8813/3   fascial
M-8814/3   infantile
M-9330/3   odontogenic (T-170.__)
M-8812/3   periosteal (T-170.__)

M------- Fibrosclerosis *(SNOMED M-49020)*
M------- Fibrosing adenomatosis *(SNOMED M-74220)*
M------- Fibrosing adenosis *(SNOMED M-74220)*
M------- Fibrosis, NOS *(SNOMED M-49000)*
M-8832/0 Fibrosis, subepidermal nodular (T-173.__)

Fibrous

M-9420/3   astrocytoma (T-191.__)
M-------   defect, metaphyseal *(SNOMED M-74940)*
M-------   dysplasia, NOS *(SNOMED M-74910)*
M-9532/0   meningioma (T-192.__)
M-8724/0   papule, nose (T-173.3)
M-------   polyp *(SNOMED M-76810)*

Fibrous histiocytoma

M-8830/0   NOS
M-8830/1   atypical
M-8830/3   malignant

Fibrous mesothelioma

M-9051/3   NOS
M-9051/0   benign
M-9051/3   malignant

Fibrous tissue

T-171.9	NOS
T-171.5	abdominal wall
T-171.3	ankle
T-171.2	antecubital space
T-171.2	arm
T-171.4	axilla
T-171.7	back
T-171.6	buttock
T-171.3	calf
T-171.0	cervical region
T-171.0	cheek
T-171.4	chest
T-171.4	chest wall
T-171.0	chin
T-171.2	elbow
T-171.0	face
T-171.2	finger
T-171.7	flank
T-171.3	foot
T-171.2	forearm
T-171.0	forehead
T-171.6	gluteal region
T-171.6	groin
T-171.2	hand
T-171.0	head
T-171.3	heel
T-171.3	hip
T-171.4	infraclavicular region
T-171.6	inguinal region
T-171.3	knee
T-171.3	leg
T-171.0	neck
T-171.6	perineum
T-171.3	popliteal space
T-171.0	pterygoid fossa
T-171.6	sacrococcygeal region
T-171.0	scalp
T-171.4	scapular region
T-171.2	shoulder
T-171.0	supraclavicular region
T-171.0	temple
T-171.3	thigh
T-171.4	thoracic wall
T-171.2	thumb
T-171.3	toe
T-171.7	trunk
T-171.5	umbilicus
T-171.2	wrist

Fibroxanthoma

M-8831/0	NOS
M-8831/1	atypical
M-8831/3	malignant

M-8831/3	Fibroxanthosarcoma
T-170.7	Fibula
T-192.2	Filum terminale

Finger

T-195.4	NOS
T-173.6	NOS (carcinoma, melanoma, nevus)
T-171.2	NOS (sarcoma, lipoma)
T-170.5	bone
T-171.2	connective tissue
T-171.2	fibrous tissue
T-171.2	muscle
T-173.6	nail
T-171.2	skeletal muscle
T-173.6	skin
T-171.2	soft tissue
T-171.2	subcutaneous tissue
T-171.2	tendon
T-171.2	tendon sheath

Flank

T-195.8	NOS
T-173.5	NOS (carcinoma, melanoma, nevus)
T-171.7	NOS (sarcoma, lipoma)
T-171.7	adipose tissue
T-171.7	connective tissue
T-171.7	fatty tissue
T-171.7	fibrous tissue
T-171.7	muscle
T-171.7	skeletal muscle
T-173.5	skin
T-171.7	soft tissue
T-171.7	subcutaneous tissue
T-171.7	tendon
T-171.7	tendon sheath

Floor of mouth

T-144.9	NOS
T-144.0	anterior
T-144.1	lateral

M-------	Florid adenosis *(SNOMED M-74260)*
M-------	Focal nodular hyperplasia *(SNOMED M-72031)*

Fold

T-148.2	aryepiglottic, NOS *(excludes Laryngeal aspect of aryepiglottic fold T-161.1)*
T-148.2	aryepiglottic, hypopharyngeal aspect
T-161.1	aryepiglottic, laryngeal aspect
T-148.2	arytenoid
T-146.2	glossopalatine

Follicular

M-8330/0	adenoma (T-193.9)
M-------	cyst, jaw *(SNOMED M-26560)*
M-9697/3	germinoblastic sarcoma
M-9692/3	germinoblastoma
M-------	keratosis, inverted *(SNOMED M-72920)*
M-9691/3	reticulolymphosarcoma

Follicular adenocarcinoma

M-8330/3	NOS (T-193.9)
M-8332/3	moderately differentiated type (T-193.9)
M-8331/3	pure follicle type (T-193.9)
M-8332/3	trabecular type (T-193.9)
M-8331/3	well differentiated type (T-193.9)

Follicular and papillary

M-8340/3	adenocarcinoma (T-193.9)
M-8340/3	carcinoma (T-193.9)
M-8340/3	carcinoma, mixed (T-193.9)

Follicular carcinoma

M-8330/3	NOS (T-193.9)
M-8332/3	moderately differentiated type (T-193.9)
M-8331/3	pure follicle type (T-193.9)
M-8332/3	trabecular type (T-193.9)
M-8331/3	well differentiated type (T-193.9)

M-9690/3	Follicular lymphoma, giant
M-9696/3	Follicular lymphoma, lymphocytic, poorly differentiated

Follicular lymphosarcoma

M-9690/3	NOS
M-9696/3	lymphoblastic
M-9691/3	mixed cell type

Follicular malignant lymphoma

M-9690/3	NOS
M-9697/3	centroblastic type
M-9692/3	centroblastic-centrocytic
M-9695/3	follicular center cell, cleaved
M-9698/3	follicular center cell, non-cleaved
M-9694/3	lymphocytic, intermediate differentiation
M-9696/3	lymphocytic, poorly differentiated
M-9693/3	lymphocytic, well differentiated
M-9691/3	mixed cell type
M-9691/3	mixed lymphocytic-histiocytic
M-9691/3	mixed small cell and large cell

Foot

T-195.5	NOS
T-173.7	NOS (carcinoma, melanoma, nevus)
T-171.3	NOS (sarcoma, lipoma)
T-171.3	adipose tissue
T-170.8	bone
T-171.3	connective tissue
T-171.3	fatty tissue
T-171.3	fibrous tissue
T-170.8	joint
T-171.3	muscle
T-170.8	phalanx
T-171.3	skeletal muscle
T-173.7	skin
T-171.3	soft tissue
T-173.7	sole
T-171.3	subcutaneous tissue
T-171.3	tendon
T-171.3	tendon sheath

M-------	Fordyce's disease *(SNOMED M-26010)*

Forearm

T-195.4	NOS
T-173.6	NOS (carcinoma, melanoma, nevus)
T-171.2	NOS (sarcoma, lipoma)
T-171.2	adipose tissue
T-170.4	bone
T-171.2	connective tissue
T-171.2	fatty tissue
T-171.2	fibrous tissue
T-171.2	muscle
T-171.2	skeletal muscle
T-173.6	skin
T-171.2	soft tissue
T-171.2	subcutaneous tissue
T-171.2	tendon
T-171.2	tendon sheath

Forehead

T-173.3	NOS
T-173.3	NOS (carcinoma, melanoma, nevus)
T-171.0	NOS (sarcoma, lipoma)
T-171.0	connective tissue
T-171.0	fibrous tissue
T-173.3	skin
T-171.0	soft tissue
T-171.0	subcutaneous tissue

T-187.1	Foreskin
T-147.3	Fornix, pharyngeal
T-184.0	Fornix, vagina

Fossa

T-195.3	ischiorectal
T-194.3	pituitary
T-171.0	pterygoid, NOS
T-148.1	pyriform
T-147.2	Rosenmüller
T-146.1	tonsillar

Fossa, cranial

T-191.9	NOS
T-191.9	anterior
T-191.9	middle
T-191.9	posterior

T-184.4	Fourchette
T-191.5	Fourth ventricle

M------- Freckle, NOS *(SNOMED M-57260)*

Frenulum

T-140.5	labii, NOS
T-141.3	linguae
T-140.5	lip, NOS
T-140.4	lower lip
T-140.3	upper lip

Frontal

T-170.0	bone
T-191.1	lobe
T-191.1	pole
T-160.4	sinus

Fundus

T-151.3	gastric
T-151.3	stomach
T-182.0	uteri

M-8004/3 Fusiform cell type, malignant tumor
M-8043/3 Fusiform cell type, small cell carcinoma

- G -

M-8153/1 G cell tumor, NOS
M-8153/3 G cell tumor, malignant

T-156.0   Gallbladder

T-171.9	Ganglia, NOS
T-191.0	Ganglia, basal

M-9490/0 Gangliocytoma
M-9505/1 Ganglioglioma
M------- Ganglion cyst *(SNOMED M-33600)*
M-9490/3 Ganglioneuroblastoma
M-9490/0 Ganglioneuroma
M-9491/0 Ganglioneuromatosis

T-184.0   Gartner's duct

Gastric *(see also Stomach)*

T-151.9	NOS
T-151.2	antrum
T-151.0	cardia
T-151.4	corpus
T-151.3	fundus
T-196.2	lymph node

M-8153/1 Gastrinoma, NOS
M-8153/3 Gastrinoma, malignant

T-171.3   Gastrocnemius muscle
T-159.9   Gastrointestinal tract, NOS

M-8480/3 Gelatinous adenocarcinoma
M-8480/3 Gelatinous carcinoma
M-9411/3 Gemistocytic astrocytoma (T-191._)
M-9411/3 Gemistocytoma (T-191._)

Genital

T-184.9	organs, female, NOS
T-187.9	organs, male, NOS
T-184.9	tract, female, NOS
T-187.9	tract, male, NOS

T-184.4	Genitalia, female, external
T-184.9	Genitourinary tract, female, NOS
T-187.9	Genitourinary tract, male, NOS

Germinoblastic sarcoma

M-9632/3	NOS
M-9632/3	diffuse
M-9697/3	follicular

M-9614/3 Germinoblastoma, diffuse
M-9692/3 Germinoblastoma, follicular
M-9064/3 Germinoma

Giant

M-8790/0	blue nevus (T-173._)
M-------	condyloma *(SNOMED M-76730)*
M-9020/0	fibroadenoma, NOS (T-174._)
M-9020/0	fibroadenoma, intracanalicular (T-174._)
M-9690/3	follicular lymphoma
M-9200/0	osteoid osteoma (T-170._)
M-8761/1	pigmented nevus (T-173._)
M-8761/3	pigmented nevus, malignant melanoma in (T-173._)
M-------	rugal hypertrophy *(SNOMED M-71330)*

Giant cell

M-8030/3	and spindle cell carcinoma
M-9384/1	astrocytoma, subependymal (T-191._)
M-8031/3	carcinoma
M-9441/3	glioblastoma (T-191._)
M-------	granuloma, central *(SNOMED M-44130)*
M-------	reparative granuloma *(SNOMED M-44110)*
M-8802/3	sarcoma *(except of Bone)*
M-9250/3	sarcoma, bone (T-170._)
M-8003/3	type, malignant tumor

Giant cell tumor

M-9230/0	chondromatous (T-170._)
M-9250/1	bone, NOS (T-170._)
M-9250/3	bone, malignant (T-170._)
M-9251/1	soft parts, NOS
M-9251/3	soft parts, malignant
M-------	tendon sheath *(SNOMED M-47830)*

M-9275/0 Gigantiform cementoma (T-170._)

Gingiva

T-143.9	NOS
T-143.1	lower
T-143.1	mandibular
T-143.0	maxillary
T-143.0	upper

M-------	Gingival cyst, NOS *(SNOMED M-26540)*
M-------	Gingival cyst, odontogenic *(SNOMED M-26540)*

T-170.4 Girdle, shoulder

Gland

T-194.0	adrenal
T-184.1	Bartholin's
T-173.2	ceruminal
T-189.3	Cowper's
T-180.0	endocervical

Gland (Cont'd)

T-194.9	endocrine, NOS
T-194.8	endocrine, multiple
T-182.0	endometrial
T-190.2	lacrimal
T-174.9	mammary
T-173.1	Meibomian
T-180.0	Nabothian
T-194.1	parathyroid
T-189.4	paraurethral
T-142.0	parotid
T-142.0	parotid, duct
T-194.4	pineal
T-194.3	pituitary
T-185.9	prostate
T-142.9	salivary, NOS *(excludes Minor salivary gland; see Introduction page xviii and note under T-142)*
T-142.2	sublingual
T-142.2	sublingual, duct
T-142.9	salivary, major, NOS
T-145.9	salivary, minor, NOS *(see Introduction page xviii and note under T-142)*
T-142.1	submandibular
T-142.1	submaxillary
T-142.1	submaxillary, duct
T-194.0	suprarenal
T-193.9	thyroid
T-189.3	urethral

T-194.8 Glands, endocrine, multiple

M-------	Glandular and stromal hyperplasia *(SNOMED M-72400)*
M-------	Glandular hyperplasia *(SNOMED M-72420)*
M-------	Glandular metaplasia *(SNOMED M-73300)*

T-187.2 Glans penis

M------- Glial heterotopia, nasal *(SNOMED M-26160)*

Glioblastoma

M-9440/3	NOS (T-191._)
M-9441/3	giant cell (T-191._)
M-9440/3	multiforme (T-191._)
M-9442/3	with sarcomatous component (T-191._)

Glioma

M-9380/3	NOS *(except Nasal glioma, SNOMED M-26160)*(T-191._)
M-9400/3	astrocytic (T-191._)
M-9380/3	malignant (T-191._)
M-9382/3	mixed (T-191._)
M-------	nasal *(SNOMED M-26160)*
M-9383/1	subependymal (T-191._)

M-9381/3 Gliomatosis cerebri (T-191._)
M-9505/1 Glioneuroma
M-9380/3 Gliosarcoma (T-191._)

T-191.0   Globus pallidus

M-8712/0 Glomangioma
M-8710/3 Glomangiosarcoma
M-8374/0 Glomerulosa cell type, adrenal cortical
              adenoma (T-194.0)
M-8710/3 Glomoid sarcoma

T-194.6   Glomus, coccygeal
T-194.6   Glomus jugulare

M-8690/1 Glomus jugulare tumor (T-194.6)
M-8711/0 Glomus tumor

T-146.2   Glossopalatine fold
T-192.0   Glossopharyngeal nerve
T-161.0   Glottis

M-8152/0 Glucagonoma, NOS (T-157._)
M-8152/3 Glucagonoma, malignant (T-157._)

Gluteal region
T-195.3   NOS
T-173.5   NOS (carcinoma, melanoma, nevus)
T-171.6   NOS (sarcoma, lipoma)
T-171.6   adipose tissue
T-171.6   connective tissue
T-171.6   fatty tissue
T-171.6   fibrous tissue
T-171.6   muscle
T-171.6   skeletal muscle
T-173.5   skin
T-171.6   soft tissue
T-171.6   subcutaneous tissue

T-171.6   Gluteus maximus muscle

M-8904/0 Glycogenic rhabdomyoma
M-8243/3 Goblet cell carcinoid

Goiter
M-------   NOS (SNOMED M-71600)
M-------   adenomatous (SNOMED M-71640)
M-------   colloid (SNOMED M-71620)
M-------   endemic (SNOMED M-71660)

M-8590/1 Gonadal stromal tumor
M-9073/1 Gonadoblastoma
M-9073/1 Gonocytoma

Grade (see Grading code, page 20)
M-___/_(1)   I
M-___/_(2)   II
M-___/_(3)   III
M-___/_(4)   IV
M-___/_(9)   Grade or differentiation not determined,
                  not stated or not applicable

Granular cell
M-8320/3   adenocarcinoma
M-8320/3   carcinoma
M-9580/0   myoblastoma, NOS
M-9580/3   myoblastoma, malignant
M-9580/0   tumor, NOS
M-9580/3   tumor, malignant

M-------   Granulation tissue type hemangioma
                  (SNOMED M-44440)
M-9930/3 Granulocytic sarcoma

Granuloma
M-------   NOS (SNOMED M-44000)
M-------   central giant cell (SNOMED M-44130)
M-------   eosinophilic, NOS (SNOMED M-44050)
M-------   eosinophilic, bone (SNOMED M-77860)
M-------   giant cell reparative (SNOMED M-44110)
M-9661/3   Hodgkin's
M-------   plasma cell (SNOMED M-43060)
M-------   pyogenic (SNOMED M-44440)
M-------   pyogenicum (SNOMED M-44440)
M-------   reticulohistiocytic (SNOMED M-77880)
M-------   sarcoid (SNOMED M-44210)

Granulosa cell
M-8620/3   carcinoma (T-183.0)
M-8620/1   tumor, NOS (T-183.0)
M-8620/3   tumor, malignant (T-183.0)

M-8621/1 Granulosa cell-theca cell tumor (T-183.0)
M-8312/3 Grawitz tumor (T-189.0)

T-151.6   Greater curvature of stomach, NOS
                  (not classifiable to T-151.0 to T-151.4)

Groin
T-195.3   NOS
T-173.5   NOS (carcinoma, melanoma, nevus)
T-171.6   NOS (sarcoma, lipoma)
T-171.6   adipose tissue
T-171.6   connective tissue
T-171.6   fatty tissue
T-171.6   fibrous tissue

Groin (Cont'd)

T-196.5	lymph node
T-173.5	skin
T-171.6	soft tissue
T-171.6	subcutaneous tissue

M-9841/3 Guglielmo's disease (T-169._)

Gum

T-143.9	NOS
T-143.1	lower
T-143.0	upper

M-8632/1 Gynandroblastoma (T-183.0)
M------- Gynecomastia *(SNOMED M-71000)*

- H -

M-9940/3 Hairy cell leukemia (T-169._)
M-8720/0 Hairy nevus (T-173._)
M-8723/0 Halo nevus (T-173._)

Hamartoma

M-------	NOS *(SNOMED M-75500)*
M-------	angiomatous lymphoid *(SNOMED M-72260)*
M-------	mesenchymal *(SNOMED M-75660)*
M-9321/0	odontogenic, central, epithelial (T-170._)
M-9321/0	odontogenic, peripheral, gingival, epithelial (T-170._)

Hand

T-195.4	NOS
T-173.6	NOS (carcinoma, melanoma, nevus)
T-171.2	NOS (sarcoma, lipoma)
T-171.2	adipose tissue
T-170.5	bone
T-171.2	connective tissue
T-171.2	fatty tissue
T-171.2	fibrous tissue
T-170.5	joint
T-171.2	muscle
T-171.2	skeletal muscle
T-170.5	phalanx
T-173.6	skin
T-171.2	soft tissue
T-171.2	subcutaneous tissue
T-171.2	tendon
T-171.2	tendon sheath

M-------	Hand-Schüller-Christian disease *(SNOMED M-77920)*
T-145.2	Hard palate
T-145.5	Hard palate and soft palate, junction

Head

T-195.0	NOS
T-173.4	NOS (carcinoma, melanoma, nevus)
T-171.0	NOS (sarcoma, lipoma)
T-171.0	adipose tissue
T-171.0	connective tissue
T-171.0	fatty tissue
T-171.0	fibrous tissue
T-196.0	lymph node
T-171.0	muscle
T-171.0	skeletal muscle
T-173.4	skin, NOS
T-171.0	soft tissue
T-171.0	subcutaneous tissue

T-157.0	Head of pancreas
T-164.1	Heart

Heel

T-195.5	NOS
T-173.7	NOS (carcinoma, melanoma, nevus)
T-171.3	NOS (sarcoma, lipoma)
T-170.8	bone
T-171.3	connective tissue
T-171.3	fibrous tissue
T-173.7	skin
T-171.3	soft tissue
T-171.3	subcutaneous tissue
T-171.3	tendon
T-171.3	tendon sheath

T-173.2 Helix

M-9535/0 Hemangioblastic meningioma (T-192._)
M-9161/1 Hemangioblastoma
M-9130/3 Hemangioendothelial sarcoma

Hemangioendothelioma

M-9130/1	NOS
M-9130/0	benign
M-9130/3	malignant

Hemangioma

M-9120/0	NOS
M-9123/0	arteriovenous
M-9131/0	capillary

Hemangioma (Cont'd)

M-9121/0	cavernous
M-------	granulation tissue type
	(SNOMED M-44440)
M-9131/0	infantile
M-9132/0	intramuscular
M-9131/0	juvenile
M-9131/0	plexiform
M-9123/0	racemose
M-8832/0	sclerosing (T-173._)
M-9131/0	simplex
M-9122/0	venous
M-9142/0	verrucous keratotic

M-------	Hemangiomatosis, NOS *(SNOMED M-76310)*
M-------	Hemangiomatosis, systemic
	(SNOMED M-76314)
M-9536/0	Hemangiopericytic meningioma (T-192._)

Hemangiopericytoma

M-9150/1	NOS
M-9150/0	benign
M-9150/3	malignant

M-9120/3	Hemangiosarcoma
M-------	Hematoma, NOS *(SNOMED M-37100)*

T-169.9	Hematopoietic system, NOS
T-191.0	Hemisphere, cerebral

M-9175/0	Hemolymphangioma
M-9140/3	Hemorrhagic sarcoma, multiple

Hepatic

T-155.0	NOS
T-156.1	bile duct
T-156.1	duct
T-153.0	flexure of colon
T-196.2	lymph node

M-8970/3	Hepatoblastoma (T-155.0)
M-8170/3	Hepatocarcinoma (T-155.0)
M-8170/0	Hepatocellular adenoma (T-155.0)

Hepatocellular carcinoma

M-8170/3	NOS (T-155.0)
M-8180/3	and bile duct carcinoma, mixed (T-155.0)
M-8180/3	and cholangiocarcinoma, combined (T-155.0)

M-8180/3	Hepatocholangiocarcinoma (T-155.0)
M-8180/0	Hepatocholangioma, benign (T-155.0)

Hepatoma

M-8170/3	NOS (T-155.0)
M-8170/0	benign (T-155.0)
M-8970/3	embryonal (T-155.0)
M-8170/3	malignant (T-155.0)

M-------	Heterotopia, NOS *(SNOMED M-26000)*
M-------	Heterotopia, nasal glial *(SNOMED M-26160)*
M-8880/0	Hibernoma

Hidradenoma

M-8400/0	NOS (T-173._)
M-8402/0	clear cell (T-173._)
M-8400/0	nodular (T-173._)
M-8405/0	papillary (T-173._)

M-8404/0	Hidrocystoma (T-173._)
M-8660/0	Hilar cell tumor (T-183.0)

Hilar lymph node

T-196.1	NOS
T-196.1	pulmonary
T-196.2	splenic

T-162.2	Hilus of lung

Hip

T-195.5	NOS
T-173.7	NOS (carcinoma, melanoma, nevus)
T-171.3	NOS (sarcoma, lipoma)
T-171.3	adipose tissue
T-170.6	bone
T-171.3	connective tissue
T-171.3	fatty tissue
T-171.3	fibrous tissue
T-170.6	joint
T-173.7	skin
T-171.3	soft tissue
T-171.3	subcutaneous tissue
T-171.3	tendon
T-171.3	tendon sheath

T-191.2	Hippocampus

M-9721/3	Histiocytic medullary reticulosis

Histiocytoma

M-8832/0	NOS (T-173._)
M-8830/0	fibrous, NOS
M-8830/1	fibrous, atypical
M-8830/3	fibrous, malignant

Histiocytosis

M-------	NOS *(SNOMED M-77800)*
M-9722/3	acute differentiated progressive
M-9720/3	malignant
M-------	sinus, with massive lymphadenopathy *(SNOMED M-77940)*
M-------	X, NOS *(SNOMED M-77910)*
M-9722/3	X, acute progressive

Hodgkin's

M-9661/3	granuloma
M-9660/3	paragranuloma
M-9662/3	sarcoma
M-9650/3	type, malignant lymphoma

Hodgkin's disease

M-9650/3	NOS
M-9653/3	lymphocytic depletion, NOS
M-9654/3	lymphocytic depletion, diffuse fibrosis
M-9655/3	lymphocytic depletion, reticular type
M-9651/3	lymphocytic predominance
M-9651/3	lymphocytic-histiocytic predominance
M-9652/3	mixed cellularity
M-9656/3	nodular sclerosis, NOS
M-9657/3	nodular sclerosis, cellular phase

T-170.4	Humerus

Hürthle cell

M-8290/3	adenocarcinoma **(T-193.9)**
M-8290/0	adenoma **(T-193.9)**
M-8290/3	carcinoma **(T-193.9)**
M-8290/0	tumor **(T-193.9)**

M-8742/2	Hutchinson's melanotic freckle **(T-173._)**
M-8742/3	Hutchinson's melanotic freckle, malignant melanoma in **(T-173._)**
M-9100/0	Hydatid mole **(T-181.9)**

Hydatidiform mole

M-9100/0	NOS **(T-181.9)**
M-9100/1	invasive **(T-181.9)**
M-9100/1	malignant **(T-181.9)**

M-9173/0	Hygroma, NOS
M-9173/0	Hygroma, cystic

T-184.0	Hymen
T-170.0	Hyoid bone

M-8052/0	Hyperkeratotic papilloma
M-8311/1	Hypernephroid tumor
M-8312/3	Hypernephroma **(T-189.0)**

Hyperplasia

M-------	NOS *(SNOMED M-72000)*
M-------	adenomatous *(SNOMED M-72420)*
M-------	adenomyomatous *(SNOMED M-72440)*
M-------	angiofollicular, benign *(SNOMED M-72260)*
M-------	atrophy-associated *(SNOMED M-72425)*
M-------	atypical *(SNOMED M-72005)*
M-------	glandular *(SNOMED M-72420)*
M-------	glandular and stromal *(SNOMED M-72400)*
M-------	lobular *(SNOMED M-72100)*
M-------	lymphoid, NOS *(SNOMED M-72200)*
M-------	nodular, NOS *(SNOMED M-72030)*
M-------	nodular focal *(SNOMED M-72031)*
M-------	papilliferous *(SNOMED M-72050)*
M-------	pseudoepitheliomatous *(SNOMED M-72090)*
M-------	stromal *(SNOMED M-72430)*
M-------	stromal and glandular *(SNOMED M-72400)*

M-------	Hyperplastic polyp *(SNOMED M-72040)*
M-------	Hyperplastic scar *(SNOMED M-49730)*
M-------	Hyperthecosis *(SNOMED M-73040)*
M-------	Hypertrophy, NOS *(SNOMED M-71000)*
M-------	Hypertrophy, giant rugal *(SNOMED M-71330)*

T-196.6	Hypogastric lymph node
T-192.0	Hypoglossal nerve
T-148.2	Hypopharyngeal aspect of aryepiglottic fold
T-148.9	Hypopharyngeal wall
T-148.9	Hypopharynx, NOS
T-148.3	Hypopharynx, posterior wall
T-194.3	Hypophysis
T-191.0	Hypothalamus

- I -

M-9962/1	Idiopathic thrombocythemia **(T-169._)**

T-153.4	Ileocecal junction
T-153.4	Ileocecal valve
T-196.2	Ileocolic lymph node
T-152.2	Ileum *(excludes Ileocecal valve T-153.4)*

Iliac

T-171.6	artery
T-196.6	lymph node
T-171.6	vein

T-171.5	Iliopsoas muscle
T-170.6	Ilium

M-9080/3	Immature teratoma

Immunoblastic

M-------	lymphadenopathy (SNOMED M-72280)
M-9612/3	lymphoma
M-9612/3	lymphosarcoma
M-9612/3	sarcoma
M-9612/3	type malignant lymphoma

M-____/2	In-situ (see Behavior code, page 20)

In-situ (see Introduction, page xiv)

M-8140/2	adenocarcinoma
M-8010/2	carcinoma, NOS
M-8070/2	carcinoma, epidermoid, NOS
M-8076/2	carcinoma, epidermoid with questionable stromal invasion (T-180._)
M-8500/2	carcinoma, intraduct
M-8520/2	carcinoma, lobular (T-174._)
M-8050/2	carcinoma, papillary
M-8070/2	carcinoma, squamous cell, NOS
M-8076/2	carcinoma, squamous cell with questionable stromal invasion (T-180._)
M-8120/2	carcinoma, transitional cell

Infantile

M-8814/3	fibrosarcoma
M-9131/0	hemangioma
M-9722/3	reticuloendotheliosis, acute
M-9071/3	type, embryonal carcinoma

Inferior

T-196.6	epigastric lymph node
T-196.2	mesenteric lymph node
T-171.5	vena cava

Infiltrating

M-8861/1	angiolipoma
M-8500/3	duct adenocarcinoma (T-174._)
M-8500/3	duct carcinoma (T-174._)
M-8541/3	duct carcinoma and Paget's disease (T-174._)

Infiltrating (Cont'd)

M-8521/3	ductular carcinoma
M-8856/0	lipoma
M-8520/3	lobular carcinoma (T-174._)

M-------	Infiltrative fasciitis (SNOMED M-76130)

Inflammatory

M-8530/3	adenocarcinoma (T-174._)
M-8530/3	carcinoma (T-174._)
M-------	polyp (SNOMED M-76820)
M-------	pseudotumor (SNOMED M-76820)

T-196.3	Infraclavicular lymph node

Infraclavicular region

T-195.1	NOS
T-173.5	NOS (carcinoma, melanoma, nevus)
T-171.4	NOS (sarcoma, lipoma)
T-171.4	adipose tissue
T-171.4	connective tissue
T-171.4	fatty tissue
T-171.4	fibrous tissue
T-196.3	lymph node
T-173.5	skin
T-171.4	soft tissue
T-171.4	subcutaneous tissue

T-196.5	Inguinal lymph node

Inguinal region

T-195.3	NOS
T-173.5	NOS (carcinoma, melanoma, nevus)
T-171.6	NOS (sarcoma, lipoma)
T-171.6	adipose tissue
T-171.6	connective tissue
T-171.6	fatty tissue
T-171.6	fibrous tissue
T-196.5	lymph node
T-173.5	skin
T-171.6	soft tissue
T-171.6	subcutaneous tissue

Inner

T-174.8	breast
T-173.1	canthus
T-160.1	ear

Inner aspect of lip

T-140.5	NOS
T-140.4	lower
T-140.3	upper

T-170.6	Innominate bone
T-196.1	Innominate lymph node
T-191.0	Insula

M-8151/0	Insulinoma, NOS (T-157._)
M-8151/3	Insulinoma, malignant (T-157._)

Intercostal

T-196.1	lymph node
T-171.4	muscle
T-171.4	nerve

Internal

T-191.0	capsule
T-145.0	cheek
T-140.5	lip, NOS
T-171.4	mammary artery
T-160.0	nose
T-180.0	os
T-188.5	urethral orifice

M-------	Internal endometriosis (SNOMED M-76510)

Interstitial cell tumor

M-8650/1	NOS
M-8650/0	benign
M-8650/3	malignant

T-170.2	Intervertebral disc
T-196.2	Intestinal lymph node
T-159.0	Intestinal tract, NOS

M-8144/3	Intestinal type adenocarcinoma (T-151.__)
M-8144/3	Intestinal type carcinoma (T-151._)

Intestine

T-159.0	NOS
T-153.9	large (excludes Rectum, NOS T-154.1 and Rectosigmoid junction T-154.0)
T-152.9	small

T-196.2	Intra-abdominal lymph nodes
T-195.2	Intra-abdominal site, NOS

Intracanalicular fibroadenoma

M-9011/0	NOS (T-174._)
M-9020/0	cellular (T-174._)
M-9020/0	giant (T-174._)

Intracranial

T-192.1	arachnoid
T-192.1	meninges
T-191.9	site

Intracystic

M-8504/0	adenoma, papillary
M-8504/2	carcinoma, non-infiltrating
M-8504/0	papilloma

M-8750/0	Intradermal nevus (T-173._)
M-8500/2	Intraduct carcinoma-in-situ

Intraductal

M-8500/2	adenocarcinoma, non-infiltrating, NOS
M-8503/2	adenocarcinoma, non-infiltrating, papillary
M-8500/2	carcinoma, NOS
M-8500/2	carcinoma, non-infiltrating, NOS
M-8503/2	carcinoma, non-infiltrating, papillary
M-8503/0	papilloma
M-8505/0	papillomatosis, NOS
M-8505/0	papillomatosis, diffuse

Intraepidermal

M-8070/2	carcinoma, NOS
M-8096/0	epithelioma, Jadassohn (T-173._)
M-8740/0	nevus (T-173._)
M-8081/2	squamous cell carcinoma, Bowen's type (T-173._)

M-____/2	Intraepithelial (see Behavior code, page 20)
M-8010/2	Intraepithelial carcinoma, NOS
M-8070/2	Intraepithelial squamous cell carcinoma

T-155.1	Intrahepatic bile duct

M-9132/0	Intramuscular hemangioma
M-8856/0	Intramuscular lipoma

T-190.0	Intraocular

M-9270/3	Intraosseous carcinoma (T-170.1)

T-196.6	Intrapelvic lymph node

T-196.1	Intrathoracic lymph node
T-195.1	Intrathoracic site, NOS

M-8890/1 Intravascular leiomyomatosis

T-161.0 Intrinsic larynx

Invasive

M-8821/1	fibroma
M-9100/1	hydatidiform mole (T-181.9)
M-9100/1	mole, NOS (T-181.9)

Inverted

M-------	follicular keratosis (SNOMED M-72920)
M-8053/0	papilloma
M-8121/1	type transitional cell papilloma

M-8724/0 Involuting nevus (T-173._)

T-190.0	Iris
T-195.3	Ischiorectal fossa
T-170.6	Ischium
T-191.0	Island of Reil
T-157.4	Islands of Langerhans

Islet cell

M-8150/3	adenocarcinoma (T-157._)
M-8150/0	adenoma (T-157._)
M-8154/3	and exocrine adenocarcinoma, mixed (T-157._)
M-8150/3	carcinoma (T-157._)
M-8150/0	tumor (T-157._)

T-157.4	Islets of Langerhans
T-182.1	Isthmus uteri

- J -

Jadassohn's

M-8780/0	blue nevus (T-173._)
M-8096/0	intraepidermal epithelioma (T-173._)
M-------	nevus sebaceus (SNOMED M-75750)

Jaw

T-195.0	NOS
T-170.1	bone, NOS
T-170.1	bone, lower

Jaw (Cont'd)

T-170.0	bone, upper
T-173.3	skin

T-152.1 Jejunum

M------- Jessner, benign lymphocytic infiltrate (SNOMED M-47250)

Joint

T-170.9	NOS
T-170.4	acromioclavicular
T-170.8	ankle
T-170.3	costovertebral
T-170.4	elbow
T-170.8	foot
T-170.5	hand
T-170.6	hip
T-170.7	knee, NOS
T-170.7	knee, lateral meniscus
T-170.7	knee, medial meniscus
T-170.4	shoulder
T-170.3	sternocostal
T-170.1	temporomandibular
T-170.5	wrist

T-196.0 Jugular lymph node

M-8690/1 Jugular paraganglioma (T-194.6)

Junction

T-154.8	anorectal
T-151.0	cardio-esophageal
T-151.0	esophagogastric
T-151.0	gastroesophageal
T-145.5	hard and soft palate
T-153.4	ileocecal
T-154.0	pelvi-rectal
T-189.1	pelvi-ureteric
T-154.0	rectosigmoid
T-180.8	squamocolumnar of cervix

M-8740/0 Junction nevus (T-173._)
M-8740/0 Junctional nevus (T-173._)
M-8740/3 Junctional nevus, malignant melanoma in (T-173._)

T-146.5	Junctional region of oropharynx
T-141.5	Junctional zone of tongue

Juvenile

M-9160/0	angiofibroma	**(T-147._)**
M-------	aponeurotic fibroma	*(SNOMED M-76150)*
M-9421/3	astrocytoma	**(T-191._)**
M-8502/3	carcinoma, breast	**(T-174._)**
M-9030/0	fibroadenoma	**(T-174._)**
M-9131/0	hemangioma	
M-8770/0	melanoma	**(T-173._)**
M-8770/0	nevus	**(T-173._)**
M-------	polyp	*(SNOMED M-75640)*
M-------	xanthogranuloma	*(SNOMED M-55380)*

Juxtacortical

M-9221/0	chondroma	**(T-170._)**
M-9221/3	chondrosarcoma	
M-9190/3	osteogenic sarcoma	**(T-170._)**
M-9190/3	osteosarcoma	**(T-170._)**

M-8361/1 Juxtaglomerular tumor **(T-189.0)**

- K -

M-9140/3 Kaposi's sarcoma
M------- Keloid *(SNOMED M-49720)*

Keratinizing type

M-8071/3	epidermoid carcinoma
M-8071/3	squamous cell carcinoma, NOS
M-8071/3	squamous cell carcinoma, large cell

M------- Keratoacanthoma, NOS *(SNOMED M-72860)*
M------- Keratocyst *(SNOMED M-26530)*

Keratosis

M-------	NOS	*(SNOMED M-72700)*
M-------	actinic	*(SNOMED M-72850)*
M-------	benign squamous	*(SNOMED M-72760)*
M-------	inverted follicular	*(SNOMED M-72920)*
M-------	obturans	*(SNOMED M-72960)*
M-------	seborrheic	*(SNOMED M-72750)*
M-------	senile	*(SNOMED M-72850)*

M-8052/0 Keratotic papilloma
M-9142/0 Keratotic verrucous hemangioma

Kidney

T-189.0	NOS

Kidney (cont'd)

T-189.0	parenchyma
T-189.1	pelvis

Knee

T-195.5	NOS
T-173.7	NOS (carcinoma, melanoma, nevus)
T-171.3	NOS (sarcoma, lipoma)
T-171.3	adipose tissue
T-171.3	connective tissue
T-171.3	fatty tissue
T-171.3	fibrous tissue
T-170.7	joint, NOS
T-170.7	joint, lateral meniscus
T-170.7	joint, medial meniscus
T-170.8	patella
T-173.7	skin
T-171.3	soft tissue
T-171.3	subcutaneous tissue
T-171.3	tendon
T-171.3	tendon sheath

M-8490/6 Krukenberg tumor **(T-183.0)**
M-9124/3 Kupffer cell sarcoma **(T-155.0)**

- L -

Labia

T-184.4	NOS
T-184.1	majora, NOS
T-184.1	majora, skin
T-184.2	minora

T-140.6	Labial commissure
T-145.1	Labial sulcus

Labium

T-184.4	NOS
T-184.1	majus
T-184.2	minus

Lacrimal

T-190.7	duct, NOS
T-190.7	duct, nasal
T-190.2	gland
T-190.7	sac

T-157.4   Langerhans, islands
T-157.4   Langerhans, islets

M-8332/3 Langhans, Wuchernde Struma (T-193.9)

T-153.9   Large bowel

Large cell carcinoma
M-8012/3 NOS
M-8072/3 epidermoid, non-keratinizing type
M-8071/3 squamous cell, keratinizing type
M-8072/3 squamous cell, non-keratinizing type

T-153.9   Large intestine *(excludes Rectum, NOS T-154.1 and Rectosigmoid junction T-154.0)*

Laryngeal
T-161.1   aspect of aryepiglottic fold
T-161.3   cartilage
T-161.0   commissure

T-148.9   Laryngopharynx

Larynx
T-161.9   NOS
T-161.3   arytenoid cartilage
T-161.3   cricoid cartilage
T-161.3   cuneiform cartilage
T-161.1   epiglottis, NOS *(excludes Anterior surface of epiglottis T-146.4)*
T-161.1   epiglottis, posterior surface
T-161.1   extrinsic
T-161.1   false cord
T-161.1   false vocal cord
T-161.0   glottis
T-161.0   intrinsic
T-161.1   laryngeal aspect of aryepiglottic fold
T-161.3   laryngeal cartilage
T-161.0   laryngeal commissure
T-161.2   subglottis
T-161.1   supraglottis
T-161.3   thyroid cartilage
T-161.0   true cord
T-161.0   true vocal cord
T-161.1   ventricular band
T-161.0   vocal cord, NOS

Lateral
T-144.1   floor of mouth
T-170.7   meniscus of knee joint
T-191.5   ventricle

Lateral wall
T-146.6   mesopharynx
T-147.2   nasopharynx
T-146.6   oropharynx
T-149.0   pharynx, NOS
T-188.2   urinary bladder

T-171.4   Latissimus dorsi muscle
T-153.2   Left colon

Leg
T-195.5   NOS
T-173.7   NOS (carcinoma, melanoma, nevus)
T-171.3   NOS (sarcoma, lipoma)
T-171.3   adipose tissue
T-170.7   bone
T-171.3   connective tissue
T-171.3   fatty tissue
T-171.3   fibrous tissue
T-196.5   lymph node
T-171.3   muscle
T-171.3   skeletal muscle
T-173.7   skin
T-171.3   soft tissue
T-171.3   subcutaneous tissue
T-171.3   tendon
T-171.3   tendon sheath

M-8891/1 Leiomyoblastoma
M-8890/0 Leiomyofibroma

Leiomyoma
M-8890/0 NOS
M-8893/0 bizarre
M-8892/1 cellular
M-8891/1 epithelioid
M-8894/0 vascular

M-8890/1 Leiomyomatosis, intravascular
M-8890/3 Leiomyosarcoma, NOS
M-8891/3 Leiomyosarcoma, epithelioid

T-190.0   Lens, crystalline

M------- Lentigo, NOS *(SNOMED M-57250)*
M-8742/2 Lentigo maligna (T-173._)
M-8742/3 Lentigo maligna melanoma (T-173._)
M-9530/3 Leptomeningeal sarcoma (T-192._)

T-151.5   Lesser curvature of stomach, NOS *(not classifiable to T-151.1 to T-151.4)*

M-9722/3 Letterer-Siwe's disease
M------- Leucokeratosis *(SNOMED M-72830)*
M------- Leucoplakia, NOS *(SNOMED M-72830)*

Leukemia (T-169._)

M-9800/3   NOS
M-9801/3   acute, NOS
M-9861/3   acute, granulocytic
M-9821/3   acute, lymphatic
M-9821/3   acute, lymphocytic
M-9821/3   acute, lymphoid
M-9891/3   acute, monocytic
M-9891/3   acute, monocytoid
M-9861/3   acute, myelocytic
M-9861/3   acute, myelogenous
M-9861/3   acute, myeloid
M-9861/3   acute, myelomonocytic
M-9866/3   acute, promyelocytic
M-9804/3   aleukemic, NOS
M-9864/3   aleukemic, granulocytic
M-9824/3   aleukemic, lymphatic
M-9824/3   aleukemic, lymphocytic
M-9824/3   aleukemic, lymphoid
M-9894/3   aleukemic, monocytic
M-9894/3   aleukemic, monocytoid
M-9864/3   aleukemic, myelogenous
M-9864/3   aleukemic, myeloid
M-9870/3   basophilic
M-9801/3   blast
M-9801/3   blastic, NOS
M-9861/3   blastic, granulocytic
M-9803/3   chronic, NOS
M-9863/3   chronic, granulocytic
M-9823/3   chronic, lymphatic
M-9823/3   chronic, lymphocytic
M-9823/3   chronic, lymphoid
M-9893/3   chronic, monocytic
M-9893/3   chronic, monocytoid
M-9863/3   chronic, myelogenous
M-9863/3   chronic, myeloid
M-9863/3   chronic, myelomonocytic
M-9810/3   compound
M-9880/3   eosinophilic
M-9860/3   granulocytic, NOS
M-9861/3   granulocytic, acute
M-9864/3   granulocytic, aleukemic
M-9861/3   granulocytic, blastic
M-9863/3   granulocytic, chronic
M-9862/3   granulocytic, subacute
M-9940/3   hairy cell
M-9890/3   histiocytic

Leukemia (T-169._) (Cont'd)

M-9820/3   lymphatic, NOS
M-9821/3   lymphatic, acute
M-9824/3   lymphatic, aleukemic
M-9823/3   lymphatic, chronic
M-9822/3   lymphatic, subacute
M-9821/3   lymphoblastic
M-9820/3   lymphocytic, NOS
M-9821/3   lymphocytic, acute
M-9824/3   lymphocytic, aleukemic
M-9823/3   lymphocytic, chronic
M-9822/3   lymphocytic, subacute
M-9820/3   lymphoid, NOS
M-9821/3   lymphoid, acute
M-9824/3   lymphoid, aleukemic
M-9823/3   lymphoid, chronic
M-9822/3   lymphoid, subacute
M-9850/3   lymphosarcoma cell **(T-169.0)**
M-9900/3   mast cell
M-9910/3   megakaryocytic
M-9910/3   megakaryocytoid
M-9810/3   mixed
M-9891/3   monoblastic
M-9890/3   monocytic, NOS
M-9891/3   monocytic, acute
M-9894/3   monocytic, aleukemic
M-9893/3   monocytic, chronic
M-9863/3   monocytic, Naegeli-type
M-9890/3   monocytic, Schilling-type
M-9892/3   monocytic, subacute
M-9890/3   monocytoid, NOS
M-9891/3   monocytoid, acute
M-9894/3   monocytoid, aleukemic
M-9893/3   monocytoid, chronic
M-9892/3   monocytoid, subacute
M-9861/3   myeloblastic
M-9863/3   myelocytic, NOS
M-9861/3   myelocytic, acute
M-9860/3   myelogenous, NOS
M-9861/3   myelogenous, acute
M-9864/3   myelogenous, aleukemic
M-9863/3   myelogenous, chronic
M-9862/3   myelogenous, subacute
M-9860/3   myeloid, NOS
M-9861/3   myeloid, acute
M-9864/3   myeloid, aleukemic
M-9863/3   myeloid, chronic
M-9862/3   myeloid, subacute
M-9860/3   myelomonocytic, NOS
M-9861/3   myelomonocytic, acute
M-9863/3   myelomonocytic, chronic
M-9863/3   Naegeli-type, monocytic
M-9865/3   neutrophilic
M-9830/3   plasma cell

Leukemia (T-169._) (Cont'd)

M-9830/3	plasmacytic
M-9825/3	prolymphocytic
M-9866/3	promyelocytic, acute
M-9890/3	Schilling-type, monocytic
M-9801/3	stem cell
M-9802/3	subacute, NOS
M-9862/3	subacute, granulocytic
M-9822/3	subacute, lymphatic
M-9822/3	subacute, lymphocytic
M-9822/3	subacute, lymphoid
M-9892/3	subacute, monocytic
M-9892/3	subacute, monocytoid
M-9862/3	subacute, myelogenous
M-9862/3	subacute, myeloid
M-9910/3	thrombocytic
M-9801/3	undifferentiated

M-9940/3 Leukemic reticuloendotheliosis

Leydig cell tumor

M-8650/1	NOS (T-186._)
M-8650/0	benign (T-186._)
M-8650/3	malignant (T-186._)

M-8631/0 Leydig-Sertoli cell tumor

Lid

T-173.1	NOS
T-173.1	lower
T-173.1	upper

Ligament

T-171.9	NOS
T-183.3	broad
T-183.5	round
T-183.4	uterine
T-183.4	uterosacral

T-190.4	Limbus of cornea
T-141.9	Lingual, NOS
T-141.6	Lingual tonsil
T-162.3	Lingula, lung

M-8142/3 Linitis plastica (T-151._)

Lip

T-140.9	NOS (excludes Skin of lip T-173.0)

Lip (Cont'd)

T-140.6	commissure
T-140.6	commissure, labial
T-140.9	external, NOS
T-140.1	external, lower
T-140.0	external, upper
T-140.5	frenulum, NOS
T-140.5	frenulum labii, NOS
T-140.4	frenulum, lower
T-140.3	frenulum, upper
T-140.5	inner aspect, NOS
T-140.4	inner aspect, lower
T-140.3	inner aspect, upper
T-140.5	internal, NOS
T-140.6	labial commissure
T-140.1	lower, NOS (excludes Skin of lower lip T-173.0)
T-140.1	lower, external
T-140.4	lower, frenulum
T-140.4	lower, inner aspect
T-140.4	lower, mucosa
T-173.0	lower, skin
T-140.1	lower, vermilion border
T-140.5	mucosa, NOS
T-140.4	mucosa, lower
T-140.3	mucosa, upper
T-173.0	skin, NOS
T-140.0	upper, NOS (excludes Skin of upper lip T-173.0)
T-140.0	upper, external
T-140.3	upper, frenulum
T-140.3	upper, inner aspect
T-140.3	upper, mucosa
T-173.0	upper, skin
T-140.0	upper, vermilion border
T-140.9	vermilion border, NOS
T-140.1	vermilion border, lower
T-140.0	vermilion border, upper

M-8670/0	Lipid cell tumor, ovary (T-183.0)
M-8324/0	Lipoadenoma
M-8881/0	Lipoblastoma
M-8881/0	Lipoblastomatosis
M-------	Lipogranuloma, NOS (SNOMED M-44040)
M-8670/0	Lipoid cell tumor, ovary (T-183.0)

Lipoma

M-8850/0	NOS
M-8881/0	fetal, NOS
M-8880/0	fetal fat cell
M-8856/0	infiltrating
M-8856/0	intramuscular
M-8857/0	spindle cell

Lipomatosis

M-------	NOS *(SNOMED M-74100)*
M-------	diffuse *(SNOMED M-74103)*
M-8881/0	fetal

Liposarcoma

M-8850/3	NOS
M-8851/3	differentiated type
M-8852/3	embryonal
M-8855/3	mixed type
M-8852/3	myxoid ·
M-8854/3	pleomorphic
M-8853/3	round cell
M-8851/3	well differentiated type

T-155.0	Liver

M-8170/0	Liver cell adenoma **(T-155.0)**
M-8170/3	Liver cell carcinoma **(T-155.0)**

Lobe

T-191.1	frontal
T-162.5	lower, bronchus
T-162.5	lower, lung
T-162.4	middle, bronchus
T-162.4	middle, lung
T-191.4	occipital
T-191.3	parietal
T-191.2	temporal
T-162.3	upper, bronchus
T-162.3	upper, lung

M-8520/3	Lobular adenocarcinoma **(T-174._)**

Lobular carcinoma

M-8520/3	NOS **(T-174._)**
M-8520/3	infiltrating **(T-174._)**
M-8520/2	in-situ **(T-174._)**
M-8520/2	non-infiltrating **(T-174._)**

M-------	Lobular hyperplasia *(SNOMED M-72100)*

T-173.2	Lobule, ear

Lower

T-143.1	alveolar mucosa
T-143.1	alveolar ridge mucosa
T-143.1	alveolus
T-174.8	breast

Lower (Cont'd)

T-143.1	gingiva
T-143.1	gum
T-174.3	inner quadrant of breast
T-170.1	jaw bone
T-173.1	lid
T-140.1	lip, NOS *(excludes Skin of lower lip T-173.0)*
T-140.1	lip, external
T-140.4	lip, frenulum
T-140.4	lip, inner aspect
T-140.4	lip, mucosa
T-173.0	lip, skin
T-140.1	lip, vermilion border
T-162.5	lobe, bronchus
T-162.5	lobe, lung
T-174.5	outer quadrant of breast
T-150.5	third of esophagus
T-182.1	uterine segment

Lower limb

T-195.5	NOS
T-173.7	NOS (carcinoma, melanoma, nevus)
T-171.3	NOS (sarcoma, lipoma)
T-171.3	adipose tissue
T-171.3	connective tissue
T-171.3	fatty tissue
T-171.3	fibrous tissue
T-170.7	long bones
T-170.7	long bones, joints
T-196.5	lymph node
T-171.3	muscle
T-171.3	skeletal muscle
T-170.8	short bones
T-170.8	short bones, joints
T-173.7	skin
T-171.3	soft tissue
T-171.3	subcutaneous tissue
T-171.3	tendon
T-171.3	tendon sheath

Lumbar

T-192.2	cord
T-196.2	lymph node
T-171.7	nerve

T-171.6	Lumbosacral plexus

Lung

T-162.9	NOS
T-162.9	bronchiole
T-162.9	bronchogenic
T-162.9	bronchus, NOS
T-162.5	bronchus, lower lobe
T-162.2	bronchus, main
T-162.4	bronchus, middle lobe
T-162.3	bronchus, upper lobe
T-162.2	carina
T-162.2	hilus
T-162.3	lingula
T-162.5	lower lobe
T-162.5	lower lobe, bronchus
T-162.2	main bronchus
T-162.4	middle lobe
T-162.4	middle lobe, bronchus
T-162.9	pulmonary, NOS
T-162.3	upper lobe
T-162.3	upper lobe, bronchus

M-8610/0	Luteinoma (T-183.0)
M-8610/0	Luteoma, NOS (T-183.0)
M-------	Luteoma, pregnancy (SNOMED M-79680)
T------	Lymph gland (see Lymph Node)

Lymph node

T-196.9	NOS
T-196.2	abdominal
T-196.2	aortic
T-196.3	arm
T-196.0	auricular
T-196.3	axilla
T-196.3	axillary
T-196.3	brachial
T-196.1	bronchial
T-196.1	bronchopulmonary
T-196.2	celiac
T-196.0	cervical
T-196.5	Cloquet
T-196.2	colic
T-196.2	common duct
T-196.3	cubital
T-196.1	diaphragmatic
T-196.6	epigastric, inferior
T-196.3	epitrochlear
T-196.1	esophageal
T-196.0	face
T-196.0	facial
T-196.5	femoral
T-196.2	gastric

Lymph node (Cont'd)

T-196.5	groin
T-196.0	head
T-196.2	hepatic
T-196.1	hilar, NOS
T-196.1	hilar, pulmonary
T-196.2	hilar, splenic
T-196.6	hypogastric
T-196.2	ileocolic
T-196.6	iliac
T-196.6	inferior epigastric
T-196.2	inferior mesenteric
T-196.3	infraclavicular
T-196.5	inguinal
T-196.5	inguinal region
T-196.1	innominate
T-196.1	intercostal
T-196.2	intestinal
T-196.2	intra-abdominal
T-196.6	intrapelvic
T-196.1	intrathoracic
T-196.0	jugular
T-196.5	leg
T-196.5	lower limb
T-196.2	lumbar
T-196.0	mandibular
T-196.1	mediastinal
T-196.2	mesenteric, NOS
T-196.2	mesenteric, inferior
T-196.2	mesenteric, superior
T-196.2	midcolic
T-196.8	multiple regions
T-196.0	neck
T-196.6	obturator
T-196.0	occipital
T-196.2	pancreatic
T-196.2	para-aortic
T-196.6	paracervical
T-196.6	parametrial
T-196.1	parasternal
T-196.0	parotid
T-196.3	pectoral
T-196.6	pelvic
T-196.2	periaortic
T-196.2	peripancreatic
T-196.5	popliteal
T-196.2	porta-hepatis
T-196.2	portal
T-196.0	preauricular
T-196.0	prelaryngeal

Lymph node (Cont'd)

T-196.6	presymphysial
T-196.0	pretracheal
T-196.1	pulmonary, NOS
T-196.1	pulmonary hilar
T-196.2	pyloric
T-196.2	retroperitoneal
T-196.0	retropharyngeal
T-196.5	Rosenmüller's
T-196.6	sacral
T-196.0	scalene
T-196.2	splenic, NOS
T-196.2	splenic hilar
T-196.3	subclavicular
T-196.5	subinguinal
T-196.0	sublingual
T-196.0	submandibular
T-196.0	submaxillary
T-196.0	submental
T-196.3	subscapular
T-196.2	superior mesenteric
T-196.0	supraclavicular
T-196.1	thoracic
T-196.5	tibial
T-196.1	tracheal
T-196.1	tracheobronchial
T-196.3	upper limb

T-196.8	Lymph nodes of multiple regions

Lymphadenopathy

M-------	angio-immunoblastic *(SNOMED M-72280)*
M-------	immunoblastic *(SNOMED M-72280)*
M-------	massive, with sinus histiocytosis *(SNOMED M-77940)*

M-9170/3	Lymphangioendothelial sarcoma
M-9170/0	Lymphangioendothelioma, NOS
M-9170/3	Lymphangioendothelioma, malignant

Lymphangioma

M-9170/0	NOS
M-9171/0	capillary
M-9172/0	cavernous
M-9173/0	cystic

M-------	Lymphangiomatosis, systemic *(SNOMED M-76414)*
M-9174/0	Lymphangiomyoma
M-9174/1	Lymphangiomyomatosis
M-9170/3	Lymphangiosarcoma

T-171.9	Lymphatic, NOS

M-9630/3	Lymphoblastic lymphoma, NOS
M-9630/3	Lymphoblastic lymphoma, diffuse

Lymphoblastic lymphosarcoma

M-9630/3	NOS
M-9630/3	diffuse
M-9696/3	follicular
M-9696/3	nodular

M-9630/3	Lymphoblastoma, NOS
M-9630/3	Lymphoblastoma, diffuse
M-------	Lymphocytic infiltrate of Jessner, benign *(SNOMED M-47250)*

Lymphocytic lymphoma *(see also Malignant lymphoma)*

M-9620/3	NOS
M-9620/3	diffuse, NOS
M-9630/3	diffuse, poorly differentiated
M-9696/3	follicular, poorly differentiated
M-9693/3	follicular, well differentiated
M-9690/3	nodular, NOS
M-9694/3	nodular, intermediate differentiation
M-9696/3	nodular, poorly differentiated
M-9693/3	nodular, well differentiated
M-9630/3	poorly differentiated, NOS

Lymphocytic lymphosarcoma

M-9620/3	NOS
M-9620/3	diffuse
M-9621/3	intermediate differentiation, NOS
M-9621/3	intermediate differentiation, diffuse
M-9694/3	intermediate differentiation, nodular

M-------	Lymphocytoma cutis, benign *(SNOMED M-72210)*
M-8082/3	Lymphoepithelial carcinoma
M-------	Lymphoepithelial lesion, benign *(SNOMED M-72240)*
M-8082/3	Lymphoepithelioma
M-9650/3	Lymphogranuloma, malignant
M-9650/3	Lymphogranulomatosis, malignant

Lymphoid

M-------	hamartoma, angiomatous *(SNOMED M-72260)*

Lymphoid (Cont'd)

M-------	hyperplasia, NOS *(SNOMED M-72200)*
M-------	polyp, NOS *(SNOMED M-76880)*
M-------	polyp, benign *(SNOMED M-76880)*

Lymphoma *(see also Malignant lymphoma)*

M-9590/3	NOS
M-9750/3	Burkitt's
M-9690/3	giant follicular
M-9612/3	immunoblastic
M-9630/3	lymphoblastic, NOS
M-9630/3	lymphoblastic, diffuse
M-9590/3	malignant, NOS
M-------	orbital *(SNOMED M-72290)*
M-9601/3	stem cell

M-------	Lymphomatoid papulosis *(SNOMED M-72230)*
M-9590/0	Lymphomatous tumor, benign
M-9611/3	Lymphoplasmacytic lymphosarcoma, diffuse
M-9970/1	Lymphoproliferative disease, chronic

Lymphosarcoma

M-9610/3	NOS
M-9850/3	cell leukemia (T-169.0)
M-9610/3	diffuse, NOS
M-9611/3	diffuse, lymphoplasmacytic
M-9611/3	diffuse, with plasmacytoid differentiation
M-9690/3	follicular, NOS
M-9696/3	follicular, lymphoblastic
M-9691/3	follicular, mixed cell type
M-9612/3	immunoblastic
M-9630/3	lymphoblastic, NOS
M-9630/3	lymphoblastic, diffuse
M-9696/3	lymphoblastic, follicular
M-9696/3	lymphoblastic, nodular
M-9620/3	lymphocytic, NOS
M-9620/3	lymphocytic, diffuse
M-9621/3	lymphocytic, intermediate differentiation, NOS
M-9621/3	lymphocytic, intermediate differentiation, diffuse
M-9694/3	lymphocytic, intermediate differentiation, nodular
M-9613/3	mixed cell type, NOS
M-9613/3	mixed cell type, diffuse
M-9691/3	mixed cell type, follicular
M-9691/3	mixed cell type, nodular
M-9690/3	nodular, NOS
M-9696/3	nodular, lymphoblastic
M-9694/3	nodular, lymphocytic, intermediate differentiation

Lymphosarcoma (Cont'd)

M-9691/3	nodular, mixed cell type
M-9631/3	prolymphocytic
M-9610/3	type, malignant lymphoma

- M -

M-8334/0	Macrofollicular adenoma (T-193.9)
M-8726/0	Magnocellular nevus (T-190.0)

T-162.2	Main bronchus
T-142.9	Major salivary gland, NOS

M-------	Malakoplakia *(SNOMED M-43180)*

Male

T-175.9	breast, NOS *(excludes Skin of breast T-173.5)*
T-187.9	genital organs, NOS
T-187.9	genital tract, NOS
T-187.9	genitourinary tract, NOS

M-8110/0	Malherbe's calcifying epithelioma (T-173.__)
M-8000/3	Malignancy
M-____/1	Malignancy, borderline *(see Behavior code, page 20)*

Malignant

M-____/6	metastatic site *(see Behavior code, page 20)*
M-____/3	primary site *(see Behavior code, page 20)*
M-____/6	secondary site *(see Behavior code, page 20)*
M-____/9	uncertain whether primary or metastatic site *(see Behavior code, page 20)*

Malignant lymphoma

M-9590/3	NOS
M-9750/3	Burkitt's type, lymphoblastic
M-9750/3	Burkitt's type, undifferentiated
M-9632/3	centroblastic type, NOS
M-9632/3	centroblastic type, diffuse
M-9697/3	centroblastic type, follicular
M-9614/3	centroblastic-centrocytic, diffuse
M-9692/3	centroblastic-centrocytic, follicular
M-9622/3	centrocytic
M-9602/3	convoluted cell type, NOS
M-9602/3	convoluted cell type, lymphoblastic

Malignant lymphoma (Cont'd)

M-9590/3	diffuse, NOS *(see also list below)*
M-9690/3	follicular, NOS *(see also list below)*
M-9615/3	follicular center cell, NOS *(see also list below)*
M-9622/3	germinocytic
M-9640/3	histiocytic, NOS *(see also list below)*
M-9650/3	Hodgkin's type
M-9612/3	immunoblastic type
M-9750/3	lymphoblastic, Burkitt's type
M-9602/3	lymphoblastic, convoluted cell type
M-9620/3	lymphocytic cell type *(see also list below)*
M-9613/3	lymphocytic-histiocytic, mixed, NOS
M-9613/3	lymphocytic-histiocytic, mixed, diffuse
M-9611/3	lymphoplasmacytoid type
M-9610/3	lymphosarcoma type
M-9613/3	mixed cell type, NOS *(see also list below)*
M-9613/3	mixed lymphocytic-histiocytic, NOS *(see also list below)*
M-9613/3	mixed small cell and large cell, NOS *(see also list below)*
M-9690/3	nodular, NOS *(see also list below)*
M-9600/3	non-Burkitt's, undifferentiated cell type
M-9591/3	non-Hodgkin's type
M-9641/3	pleomorphic cell type, histiocytic
M-9640/3	reticulum cell type
M-9601/3	stem cell type
M-9750/3	undifferentiated, Burkitt's type
M-9600/3	undifferentiated cell type, NOS
M-9600/3	undifferentiated cell type, non-Burkitt's

Malignant lymphoma, diffuse

M-9590/3	NOS
M-9632/3	centroblastic type
M-9614/3	centroblastic-centrocytic
M-9615/3	follicular center cell, NOS
M-9623/3	follicular center cell, cleaved
M-9633/3	follicular center cell, non-cleaved
M-9640/3	histiocytic
M-9621/3	lymphocytic, intermediate differentiation
M-9630/3	lymphocytic, poorly differentiated
M-9620/3	lymphocytic, well differentiated
M-9611/3	lymphocytic with plasmacytoid differentiation
M-9613/3	mixed cell type
M-9613/3	mixed lymphocytic-histiocytic
M-9613/3	mixed small cell and large cell

Malignant lymphoma, follicular

M-9690/3	NOS
M-9697/3	centroblastic type
M-9692/3	centroblastic-centrocytic
M-9695/3	follicular center cell, cleaved

Malignant lymphoma, follicular (Cont'd)

M-9698/3	follicular center cell, non-cleaved
M-9694/3	lymphocytic, intermediate differentiation
M-9696/3	lymphocytic, poorly differentiated
M-9693/3	lymphocytic, well differentiated
M-9691/3	mixed cell type
M-9691/3	mixed lymphocytic-histiocytic
M-9691/3	mixed small cell and large cell

Malignant lymphoma, follicular center cell

M-9615/3	NOS
M-9623/3	cleaved, NOS
M-9623/3	cleaved, diffuse
M-9695/3	cleaved, follicular
M-9615/3	diffuse, NOS
M-9633/3	non-cleaved, NOS
M-9633/3	non-cleaved, diffuse
M-9698/3	non-cleaved, follicular

Malignant lymphoma, histiocytic

M-9640/3	NOS
M-9640/3	diffuse
M-9642/3	nodular
M-9641/3	pleomorphic cell type

Malignant lymphoma, lymphocytic

M-9620/3	cell type
M-9621/3	intermediate differentiation, NOS
M-9621/3	intermediate differentiation, diffuse
M-9694/3	intermediate differentiation, follicular
M-9694/3	intermediate differentiation, nodular
M-9630/3	poorly differentiated, NOS
M-9630/3	poorly differentiated, diffuse
M-9696/3	poorly differentiated, follicular
M-9696/3	poorly differentiated, nodular
M-9620/3	well differentiated, NOS
M-9620/3	well differentiated, diffuse
M-9693/3	well differentiated, follicular
M-9693/3	well differentiated, nodular
M-9611/3	with plasmacytoid differentiation, diffuse

Malignant lymphoma, mixed cell type

M-9613/3	NOS
M-9613/3	diffuse
M-9691/3	follicular
M-9691/3	nodular

Malignant lymphoma, mixed lymphocytic-histiocytic

M-9613/3 NOS
M-9613/3 diffuse
M-9691/3 follicular
M-9691/3 nodular

Malignant lymphoma, mixed small cell and large cell

M-9613/3 NOS
M-9613/3 diffuse
M-9691/3 follicular
M-9691/3 nodular

Malignant lymphoma, nodular

M-9690/3 NOS
M-9642/3 histiocytic
M-9694/3 lymphocytic, intermediate differentiation
M-9696/3 lymphocytic, poorly differentiated
M-9693/3 lymphocytic, well differentiated
M-9691/3 mixed cell type
M-9691/3 mixed lymphocytic-histiocytic
M-9691/3 mixed small cell and large cell

T-171.4 Mammary artery, internal
M------- Mammary duct ectasia *(SNOMED M-32100)*
T-174.9 Mammary gland
T-170.1 Mandible
T-143.1 Mandibular gingiva
T-196.0 Mandibular lymph node

M-8670/0 Masculinovoblastoma (T-183.0)

T-171.0 Masseter muscle

Mast cell

M-9741/3 disease, systemic tissue
M-9900/3 leukemia (T-169.__)
M-9740/3 sarcoma
M-9740/1 tumor, NOS
M-9740/3 tumor, malignant

M-9740/1 Mastocytoma, NOS
M-9740/3 Mastocytoma, malignant
M-9741/3 Mastocytosis, malignant

T-160.1 Mastoid antrum

M-9080/0 Mature teratoma

T-170.0 Maxilla

Maxillary

T-160.2 antrum
T-143.0 gingiva
T-160.2 sinus

T-173.2 Meatus, external auditory
T-152.3 Meckel's diverticulum *(site of neoplasm)*
T-170.7 Medial meniscus of knee joint
T-171.2 Median nerve
T-196.1 Mediastinal lymph node

Mediastinum

T-164.9 NOS
T-164.2 anterior
T-164.3 posterior

T-194.0 Medulla, adrenal
T-191.7 Medulla oblongata

Medullary

M-8510/3 adenocarcinoma
M-8510/3 carcinoma, NOS
M-8511/3 carcinoma with amyloid stroma (T-193.9)
M-8512/3 carcinoma with lymphoid stroma (T-174.__)
M-9721/3 histiocytic reticulosis

M-9470/3 Medulloblastoma, NOS (T-191.6)
M-9471/3 Medulloblastoma, desmoplastic (T-191.6)
M-9501/3 Medulloepithelioma, NOS
M-9502/3 Medulloepithelioma, teratoid
M-9472/3 Medullomyoblastoma (T-191.6)

Megakaryocytic

M-9910/3 leukemia (T-169.__)
M-9961/1 myelosclerosis (T-169.1)
M-9920/3 myelosis (T-169.__)

M-9910/3 Megakaryocytoid leukemia (T-169.__)

T-173.1 Meibomian gland

M-9363/0 Melanoameloblastoma (T-170.__)
M-8720/3 Melanocarcinoma
M-8726/0 Melanocytoma, eyeball (T-190.0)

Melanoma

M-8720/3 NOS
M-8730/3 amelanotic
M-8722/3 balloon cell
M-8771/3 epithelioid cell

Melanoma (cont'd)

M-8775/3	epithelioid and spindle cell, mixed
M-8770/0	juvenile
M-8742/3	lentigo maligna (T-173._)
M-8720/3	malignant, NOS
M-8761/3	malignant, in giant pigmented nevus (T-173._)
M-8742/3	malignant, in Hutchinson's melanotic freckle (T-173._)
M-8740/3	malignant, in junctional nevus (T-173._)
M-8741/3	malignant, in precancerous melanosis (T-173._)
M-8721/3	nodular
M-8772/3	spindle cell, NOS
M-8773/3	spindle cell, type A (T-190.0)
M-8774/3	spindle cell, type B (T-190.0)
M-8775/3	spindle cell and epithelioid cell, mixed
M-8743/3	superficial spreading

M-8720/3	Melanosarcoma, NOS
M-8771/3	Melanosarcoma, epithelioid cell

Melanosis

M-------	congenital (SNOMED M-25110)
M-8741/2	precancerous, NOS (T-173._)
M-8741/3	precancerous, malignant melanoma in (T-173._)

Melanotic

M-8742/2	freckle, Hutchinson's (T-173._)
M-8742/3	freckle, Hutchinson's, malignant melanoma in (T-173._)
M-9363/0	neuroectodermal tumor
M-9541/0	neurofibroma
M-9363/0	progonoma

T-181.9	Membranes, fetal

M-9530/3	Meningeal sarcoma (T-192._)
M-9539/3	Meningeal sarcomatosis (T-192._)

Meninges

T-192.1	NOS
T-192.1	cerebral
T-192.1	cranial
T-192.1	intracranial
T-192.3	spinal

Meningioma (T-192._)

M-9530/0	NOS
M-9535/0	angioblastic
M-9534/0	angiomatous
M-9531/0	endotheliomatous
M-9532/0	fibroblastic
M-9532/0	fibrous
M-9535/0	hemangioblastic
M-9536/0	hemangiopericytic
M-9530/3	malignant
M-9531/0	meningotheliomatous
M-9537/0	mixed
M-9538/1	papillary
M-9533/0	psammomatous
M-9531/0	syncytial
M-9537/0	transitional

M-9530/1	Meningiomas, multiple (T-192._)
M-9530/1	Meningiomatosis, NOS (T-192._)
M-9530/1	Meningiomatosis, diffuse (T-192._)
M-9530/3	Meningothelial sarcoma (T-192._)
M-9531/0	Meningotheliomatous meningioma (T-192._)

T-170.7	Meniscus, lateral of knee joint
T-170.7	Meniscus, medial of knee joint

Mesenchymal

M-9240/3	chondrosarcoma
M-------	hamartoma (SNOMED M-75660)
M-8962/3	nephroblastoma (T-189.0)
M-8990/3	sarcoma, mixed
M-8800/3	tumor, malignant
M-8990/1	tumor, mixed

Mesenchymoma

M-8990/1	NOS
M-8990/0	benign
M-8990/3	malignant

T-171.5	Mesenteric artery

Mesenteric lymph node

T-196.2	NOS
T-196.2	inferior
T-196.2	superior

T-158.8	Mesentery
T-158.8	Mesoappendix

M-8960/1	Mesoblastic nephroma

T-158.8   Mesocolon

M-8951/3   Mesodermal mixed tumor
M-9110/3   Mesometanephric carcinoma

Mesonephric
M-9110/3   adenocarcinoma
M-9110/0   adenoma
M-9110/1   tumor

M-8310/3   Mesonephroid type clear cell adenocarcinoma

Mesonephroma
M-9110/3   NOS
M-9110/0   benign
M-9110/3   malignant

Mesopharynx
T-146.9   NOS
T-146.6   lateral wall
T-146.7   posterior wall

M-9050/3   Mesothelial sarcoma

Mesothelioma
M-9050/3   NOS
M-9050/0   benign
M-9053/3   biphasic type, NOS
M-9053/0   biphasic type, benign
M-9053/3   biphasic type, malignant
M-9052/3   epithelioid, NOS
M-9052/0   epithelioid, benign
M-9052/3   epithelioid, malignant
M-9051/3   fibrous, NOS
M-9051/0   fibrous, benign
M-9051/3   fibrous, malignant
M-9050/3   malignant

T-183.3   Mesovarium
T-170.5   Metacarpal bone

M-------   Metaphyseal fibrous defect
           (SNOMED M-74940)

Metaplasia
M-------   NOS *(SNOMED M-73000)*
M-------   glandular *(SNOMED M-73300)*
M-------   myeloid *(SNOMED M-73500)*
M-------   squamous *(SNOMED M-73220)*

M-------   Metaplastic polyp *(SNOMED M-72040)*

Metastatic
M-8140/6   adenocarcinoma, NOS
M-8010/6   carcinoma, NOS
M-8000/6   neoplasm
M-8490/6   signet ring cell carcinoma
M-8000/6   tumor

M-____/6   Metastatic site, malignant *(see Behavior code, page 20)*

T-170.8   Metatarsal bone

M-8095/3   Metatypical carcinoma (T-173._)
M-8333/0   Microfollicular adenoma (T-193.9)
M-8076/3   Micro-invasive squamous cell carcinoma
           (T-180._)
M-9710/3   Microglioma

T-191.7   Midbrain
T-196.2   Midcolic lymph node

Middle
T-191.9   cranial fossa
T-160.1   ear
T-162.4   lobe, bronchus
T-162.4   lobe, lung
T-150.4   third of esophagus

T-174.8   Midline of breast
T-141.1   Midline of tongue
T-145.9   Minor salivary gland, NOS *(see Introduction page xviii and note under T-142)*

Mixed
M-8281/0   acidophil-basophil adenoma (T-194.3)
M-8281/3   acidophil-basophil carcinoma (T-194.3)
M-8560/3   adenocarcinoma and epidermoid carcinoma
M-8560/3   adenocarcinoma and squamous cell
           carcinoma
M-8094/3   basal-squamous cell carcinoma (T-173._)
M-8281/0   basophil-acidophil adenoma (T-194.3)
M-8281/3   basophil-acidophil carcinoma (T-194.3)
M-8180/3   bile duct and hepatocellular carcinoma
           (T-155.0)
M-8323/3   cell adenocarcinoma
M-8323/0   cell adenoma
M-8375/0   cell type, adrenal cortical adenoma
           (T-194.0)
M-9081/3   embryonal carcinoma and teratoma
M-8560/3   epidermoid carcinoma and adenocarcinoma
M-8775/3   epithelioid and spindle cell melanoma
M-8154/3   exocrine and islet cell adenocarcinoma
           (T-157._)

Mixed (Cont'd)

M-8340/3   follicular and papillary carcinoma **(T-193.9)**

M-9382/3   glioma **(T-191._)**

M-8180/3   hepatocellular and bile duct carcinoma
         (T-155.0)

M-8154/3   islet cell and exocrine adenocarcinoma
         (T-157._)

M-9810/3   leukemia **(T-169._)**

M-9537/0   meningioma **(T-192._)**

M-8990/3   mesenchymal sarcoma

M-8990/1   mesenchymal tumor

M-8951/3   mesodermal tumor

M-8950/3   Müllerian tumor

M-9382/3   oligo-astrocytoma **(T-191._)**

M-8340/3   papillary and follicular carcinoma **(T-193.9)**

M-8775/3   spindle cell and epithelioid cell melanoma

M-8560/3   squamous cell carcinoma and
         adenocarcinoma

M-8094/3   squamous-basal cell carcinoma **(T-173._)**

M-9081/3   teratoma and embryonal carcinoma

M-8855/3   type liposarcoma

M-8902/3   type rhabdomyosarcoma

Mixed tumor

M-8940/0   NOS

M-8940/3   malignant, NOS

M-8940/0   salivary gland type, NOS

M-8940/3   salivary gland type, malignant

M-____/.(3) Moderately differentiated *(see Grading code, page 20)*

M-____/.(3) Moderately well differentiated *(see Grading code, page 20)*

M-8332/3 Moderately differentiated type, follicular
         adenocarcinoma **(T-193.9)**

M-8332/3 Moderately differentiated type, follicular
         carcinoma **(T-193.9)**

Mole

M-9100/0   hydatid **(T-181.9)**

M-9100/0   hydatidiform, NOS **(T-181.9)**

M-9100/1   hydatidiform, invasive **(T-181.9)**

M-9100/1   hydatidiform, malignant **(T-181.9)**

M-9100/1   invasive, NOS **(T-181.9)**

M-------- Molluscum contagiosum *(SNOMED M-76660)*

M-------- Molluscum sebaceum *(SNOMED M-72860)*

M-8146/0 Monomorphic adenoma

M-9731/1 Monostotic myeloma

T-184.4   Mons pubis

T-184.4   Mons veneris

M-9481/3 Monstrocellular sarcoma **(T-191._)**

M-8092/3 Morphea type, basal cell carcinoma **(T-173._)**

Mouth

T-145.9   NOS

T-144.9   floor, NOS

T-144.0   floor, anterior

T-144.1   floor, lateral

T-145.5   roof

T-145.1   vestibule

M-8481/3 Mucin-producing adenocarcinoma

M-8481/3 Mucin-producing carcinoma

M-8481/3 Mucin-secreting adenocarcinoma

M-8481/3 Mucin-secreting carcinoma

Mucinous

M-8480/3   adenocarcinoma

M-9015/0   adenofibroma **(T-183.0)**

M-8480/0   adenoma

M-8480/3   carcinoma

M-8470/3   cystadenocarcinoma, NOS **(T-183.0)**

M-8471/3   cystadenocarcinoma, papillary **(T-183.0)**

M-9015/0   cystadenofibroma **(T-183.0)**

M-8470/0   cystoma **(T-183.0)**

Mucinous cystadenoma

M-8470/0   NOS **(T-183.0)**

M-8470/1   borderline malignancy **(T-183.0)**

M-8471/0   papillary, NOS **(T-183.0)**

M-8471/1   papillary, borderline malignancy **(T-183.0)**

M-8243/3 Mucocarcinoid tumor, malignant

M-------- Mucocele *(SNOMED M-33200)*

M-8430/3 Mucoepidermoid carcinoma

M-8430/1 Mucoepidermoid tumor

Mucoid

M-8480/3   adenocarcinoma

M-8480/3   carcinoma

M-8300/3   cell adenocarcinoma **(T-194.3)**

M-8300/0   cell adenoma **(T-194.3)**

Mucosa

T-143.9   alveolar, NOS

T-143.1   alveolar, lower

T-143.0   alveolar, upper

T-143.9   alveolar ridge, NOS

T-143.1   alveolar ridge, lower

T-143.0   alveolar ridge, upper

Mucosa (Cont'd)

T-145.0	buccal
T-145.0	cheek
T-140.5	lip, NOS
T-140.4	lip, lower
T-140.3	lip, upper
T-160.0	nasal
T-145.9	oral

M-8480/3	Mucous adenocarcinoma
M-8480/3	Mucous carcinoma
M-8950/3	Müllerian mixed tumor
M-8091/3	Multicentric basal cell carcinoma (T-173._)

Multiple

M-8360/1	adenomas, endocrine
M-8221/0	adenomatous polyps
M-9140/3	hemorrhagic sarcoma
M-9530/1	meningiomas (T-192._)
M-9730/3	myeloma
M-9540/1	neurofibromatosis
M-8221/0	polyposis
M-8221/0	polyps, adenomatous

T-194.8	Multiple endocrine glands
T-196.8	Multiple regions, lymph nodes

Muscle

T-171.9	NOS
T-171.5	abdomen
T-171.5	abdominal wall
T-171.2	arm
T-171.7	back
T-171.2	biceps brachii
T-171.3	biceps femoris
T-171.2	brachialis
T-171.6	buttock
T-171.3	calf
T-171.4	chest wall
T-171.2	coracobrachialis
T-171.2	deltoideus
T-190.1	extra-ocular
T-171.0	face
T-171.2	finger
T-171.7	flank
T-171.3	foot
T-171.2	forearm
T-171.3	gastrocnemius
T-171.6	gluteus maximus
T-171.2	hand
T-171.0	head
T-171.5	iliopsoas

Muscle (Cont'd)

T-171.4	intercostal
T-171.4	latissimus dorsi
T-171.3	leg
T-171.0	masseter
T-171.0	neck
T-171.4	pectoralis major
T-171.6	pelvis
T-171.6	perineum
T-171.5	psoas
T-171.3	quadriceps femoris
T-171.5	rectus abdominis
T-171.6	sacrococcygeal region
T-171.0	scalp
T-171.2	shoulder
T-171.9	skeletal, NOS
T-171.0	sternocleidomastoid
T-171.3	thigh
T-171.4	thoracic wall
T-171.4	thorax
T-171.2	thumb
T-171.3	toe
T-171.4	trapezius
T-171.2	triceps brachii
T-171.7	trunk

M-------	Musculo-aponeurotic fibromatosis (SNOMED M-76150)
M-9700/3	Mycosis fungoïdes
M-------	Myelofibrosis (SNOMED M-49000)
M-------	Myeloid metaplasia (SNOMED M-73500)
M-9930/3	Myeloid sarcoma
M-8870/0	Myelolipoma

Myeloma

M-9730/3	NOS
M-9731/1	monostotic
M-9730/3	multiple
M-9730/3	plasma cell
M-9730/3	plasmacytic
M-9731/1	solitary

M-9730/3	Myelomatosis
M-9960/1	Myeloproliferative disease, chronic (T-169._)
M-9930/3	Myelosarcoma

Myelosclerosis

M-------	NOS (SNOMED M-49020)
M-9961/1	megakaryocytic (T-169.1)
M-9961/1	with myeloid metaplasia (T-169.1)

Myelosis

M-9860/3 NOS (T-169._)
M-9861/3 acute, NOS (T-169._)
M-9841/3 acute erythremic (T-169._)
M-9864/3 aleukemic (T-169._)
M-9863/3 chronic (T-169._)
M-9840/3 erythremic, NOS (T-169._)
M-9841/3 erythremic, acute (T-169._)
M-9920/3 megakaryocytic (T-169._)
M-9862/3 subacute (T-169._)

M-9580/0 Myoblastoma, granular cell, NOS
M-9580/3 Myoblastoma, granular cell, malignant

T-164.1 Myocardium

M-8982/0 Myoepithelial tumor
M-8982/0 Myoepithelioma
M-8890/0 Myofibroma
M-8895/0 Myoma

T-182.0 Myometrium

M-8895/3 Myosarcoma
M-8931/1 Myosis, stromal, NOS (T-182.0)
M-8931/1 Myosis, stromal, endolymphatic (T-182.0)
M------- Myositis ossificans, NOS (SNOMED M-73410)
M-8811/0 Myxofibroma, NOS
M-9320/0 Myxofibroma, odontogenic (T-170._)
M-8811/0 Myxoid fibroma
M-8852/3 Myxoid liposarcoma
M-8852/0 Myxolipoma
M-8852/3 Myxoliposarcoma
M-8840/0 Myxoma, NOS
M-9320/0 Myxoma, odontogenic (T-170._)
M-9394/1 Myxopapillary ependymoma (T-191._)
M-8840/3 Myxosarcoma

- N -

T-180.0 Nabothian gland
T-173.6 Nail, finger
T-173.7 Nail, toe
T-160.0 Naris

Nasal
T-170.0 bone
T-160.0 cartilage

Nasal (Cont'd)
T-160.0 cavity (excludes Nose, NOS T-195.0)
T-190.7 lacrimal duct
T-160.0 mucosa
T-160.0 septum, NOS (excludes Posterior margin of nasal septum T-147.3)
T-147.3 septum, posterior margin
T-160.9 sinus, accessory
T-160.0 turbinate

M------- Nasal glial heterotopia (SNOMED M-26160)
M------- Nasal glioma (SNOMED M-26160)

T-190.7 Nasal lacrimal duct
T-190.7 Nasolacrimal duct

M------- Nasopalatine duct cyst (SNOMED M-26600)

T-147.3 Nasopharyngeal surface, soft palate
T-147.9 Nasopharyngeal wall

Nasopharynx
T-147.9 NOS
T-147.3 anterior wall
T-147.2 lateral wall
T-147.1 posterior wall
T-147.0 roof
T-147.0 superior wall

Neck
T-195.0 NOS
T-173.4 NOS (carcinoma, melanoma, nevus)
T-171.0 NOS (sarcoma, lipoma)
T-171.0 adipose tissue
T-171.0 connective tissue
T-171.0 fatty tissue
T-171.0 fibrous tissue
T-196.0 lymph node
T-171.0 muscle
T-171.0 skeletal muscle
T-173.4 skin
T-171.0 soft tissue
T-171.0 subcutaneous tissue
T-171.0 tendon
T-171.0 tendon sheath

T-188.5 Neck of bladder

M------- Necrosis, fat (SNOMED M-54110)

Neoplasm
M-8000/1 NOS
M-8000/0 benign

Neoplasm (Cont'd)
M-8000/3	malignant
M-8000/9	malignant, uncertain whether primary or metastatic
M-8000/6	metastatic
M-8000/6	secondary
M-8000/1	uncertain whether benign or malignant

Nephroblastoma
M-8960/3	NOS (T-189.0)
M-8961/3	epithelial (T-189.0)
M-8962/3	mesenchymal (T-189.0)

M-8960/1 Nephroma, mesoblastic

Nerve
T-171.9	NOS
T-192.0	abducens
T-192.0	accessory, NOS
T-192.0	accessory, spinal
T-192.0	acoustic
T-171.2	brachial
T-192.0	cranial
T-192.0	facial
T-171.3	femoral
T-192.0	glossopharyngeal
T-192.0	hypoglossal
T-171.4	intercostal
T-171.7	lumbar
T-171.2	median
T-171.3	obturator
T-192.0	oculomotor
T-192.0	olfactory
T-192.0	optic
T-171.9	peripheral, NOS
T-171.2	radial
T-171.6	sacral
T-171.3	sciatic
T-171.9	spinal, NOS
T-192.0	trigeminal
T-192.0	trochlear
T-171.2	ulnar
T-192.0	vagus

Nervous system
T-192.9	NOS
T-171.9	autonomic
T-192.9	central
T-171.9	parasympathetic
T-171.9	sympathetic

M-8150/0	Nesidioblastoma (T-157._)
M-9560/0	Neurilemmoma, NOS
M-9560/3	Neurilemmoma, malignant
M-9560/3	Neurilemmosarcoma
M-9560/0	Neurinoma
M-9560/1	Neurinomatosis
M-9505/1	Neuroastrocytoma
M-9500/3	Neuroblastoma, NOS
M-9522/3	Neuroblastoma, olfactory (T-160._)
M-9506/0	Neurocytoma
M-9363/0	Neuroectodermal tumor, melanotic
M-9503/3	Neuroepithelioma, NOS
M-9523/3	Neuroepithelioma, olfactory (T-160._)

Neurofibroma
M-9540/0	NOS
M-9541/0	melanotic
M-9550/0	plexiform

M-9540/1	Neurofibromatosis, NOS
M-9540/1	Neurofibromatosis, multiple
M-9540/3	Neurofibrosarcoma
M-9540/3	Neurogenic sarcoma
M-9520/3	Neurogenic tumor, olfactory

Neuroma
M-9570/0	NOS
M-9560/0	acoustic (T-192.0)
M-------	amputation (SNOMED M-49770)
M-9550/0	plexiform
M-------	traumatic (SNOMED M-49770)

M-8725/0	Neuronevus (T-173._)
M-9540/3	Neurosarcoma
M-8720/3	Nevocarcinoma
M-------	Nevoxanthoendothelioma (SNOMED M-55380)

Nevus
M-8720/0	NOS (T-173._)
M-8730/0	achromic (T-173._)
M-------	araneus (SNOMED M-76330)
M-8722/0	balloon cell (T-173._)
M-8780/0	blue, NOS (T-173._)
M-8790/0	blue, cellular (T-173._)
M-8790/0	blue, giant (T-173._)
M-8780/0	blue, Jadassohn's (T-173._)
M-8780/3	blue, malignant (T-173._)
M-8760/0	compound (T-173._)
M-8750/0	dermal (T-173._)
M-8760/0	dermal and epidermal (T-173._)

Nevus (Cont'd)

M-8770/0	epithelioid and spindle cell (T-173._)
M-8770/0	epithelioid cell (T-173._)
M-------	flammeus (SNOMED M-75540)
M-8761/1	giant pigmented (T-173._)
M-8761/3	giant pigmented, malignant melanoma in (T-173._)
M-8720/0	hairy (T-173._)
M-8723/0	halo (T-173._)
M-8750/0	intradermal (T-173._)
M-8740/0	intraepidermal (T-173._)
M-8724/0	involuting (T-173._)
M-8780/0	Jadassohn's, blue (T-173._)
M-------	Jadassohn's, sebaceus (SNOMED M-75750)
M-8740/0	junction (T-173._)
M-8740/0	junctional (T-173._)
M-8740/3	junctional, malignant melanoma in
M-8770/0	juvenile (T-173._)
M-8726/0	magnocellular (T-190.0)
M-8730/0	non-pigmented (T-173._)
M-8720/0	pigmented, NOS (T-173._)
M-------	portwine (SNOMED M-75540)
M-------	sanguineous (SNOMED M-75540)
M-------	sebaceus, Jadassohn's (SNOMED M-75750)
M-------	spider (SNOMED M-76330)
M-8770/0	spindle cell (T-173._)
M-8770/0	spindle cell and epithelioid cell (T-173._)
M-------	spongy, mucosa (SNOMED M-75710)
M-------	strawberry (SNOMED M-75540)
M-------	unius lateris (SNOMED M-75740)
M-------	vascular (SNOMED M-75540)
M-------	verrucosus (SNOMED M-75740)

T-174.0   Nipple

M-9990/0 No microscopic confirmation; clinically benign tumor

M-9990/3 No microscopic confirmation; clinically malignant tumor (cancer)

M-9990/6 No microscopic confirmation; clinically metastatic tumor (cancer)

M-9990/1 No microscopic confirmation; clinically tumor, NOS

T------   Node (see Lymph Node)

Nodular

M-------	fasciitis (SNOMED M-76130)
M-8400/0	hydradenoma (T-173._)
M-------	hyperplasia, NOS (SNOMED M-72030)
M-------	hyperplasia, focal (SNOMED M-72031)
M-9690/3	lymphoma, lymphocytic, NOS
M-9694/3	lymphoma, lymphocytic, intermediate differentiation

Nodular (Cont'd)

M-9696/3	lymphoma, lymphocytic, poorly differentiated
M-9693/3	lymphoma, lymphocytic, well differentiated
M-9690/3	lymphosarcoma, NOS
M-9696/3	lymphosarcoma, lymphoblastic
M-9694/3	lymphosarcoma, lymphocytic, intermediate differentiation
M-9691/3	lymphosarcoma, mixed cell type
M-9690/3	malignant lymphoma, NOS (See also Malignant lymphoma, nodular)
M-8721/3	melanoma
M-9691/3	reticulolymphosarcoma
M-9642/3	reticulosarcoma
M-8832/0	subepidermal fibrosis (T-173._)
M-------	tenosynovitis (SNOMED M-47830)

M-8242/1 Non-argentaffin carcinoid tumor, NOS

M-8242/3 Non-argentaffin carcinoid tumor, malignant

M-9600/3 Non-Burkitt's malignant lymphoma, undifferentiated cell type

M-8693/1 Nonchromaffin paraganglioma, NOS

M-8693/3 Nonchromaffin paraganglioma, malignant

Nonencapsulated sclerosing

M-8350/3 adenocarcinoma (T-193.9)

M-8350/3 carcinoma (T-193.9)

M-8350/3 tumor (T-193.9)

M-9591/3 Non-Hodgkin's type, malignant lymphoma

M-____/2 Non-infiltrating (see Behavior code, page 20)

Non-infiltrating

M-8500/2 adenocarcinoma, intraductal, NOS

M-8503/2 adenocarcinoma, intraductal, papillary

M-8504/2 carcinoma, intracystic

M-8500/2 carcinoma, intraductal, NOS

M-8503/2 carcinoma, intraductal, papillary

M-8520/2 carcinoma, lobular (T-174._)

M-8501/2 comedocarcinoma (T-174._)

M-____/2 Non-invasive (see Behavior code, page 20)

Non-keratinizing type

M-8072/3 epidermoid carcinoma, large cell

M-8073/3 epidermoid carcinoma, small cell

M-8072/3 squamous cell carcinoma, NOS

M-8072/3 squamous cell carcinoma, large cell

M-8073/3 squamous cell carcinoma, small cell

M-9722/3 Non-lipid reticuloendotheliosis

M------- Non-ossifying fibroma (SNOMED M-74940)

M-8730/0 Non-pigmented nevus (T-173._)

Nose

T-195.0	NOS
T-173.3	ala nasi
T-170.0	bone
T-160.0	cartilage
T-147.3	choana
T-173.3	external
T-160.0	internal
T-160.0	mucosa
T-160.0	naris
T-170.0	nasal bone
T-160.0	nasal cavity
T-160.0	nostril
T-160.0	septum, NOS
T-147.3	septum, posterior margin
T-173.3	skin
T-160.0	turbinate
T-160.0	vestibule

T-160.0	Nostril
T-170.2	Nucleus pulposus

- O -

M-8042/3	Oat cell carcinoma (T-162._)

T-196.6	Obturator lymph node
T-171.3	Obturator nerve

Occipital

T-170.0	bone
T-191.4	lobe
T-196.0	lymph node
T-191.4	pole

T-192.0	Oculomotor nerve

M-9311/0	Odontoameloblastoma (T-170._)

Odontogenic

M-9300/0	adenomatoid tumor (T-170._)
M-9270/3	carcinoma (T-170._)
M-9321/0	fibroma, NOS (T-170._)
M-------	fibroma, peripheral (SNOMED M-76850)
M-9330/3	fibrosarcoma (T-170._)

Odontogenic (Cont'd)

M-9321/0	hamartoma, central, epithelial (T-170._)
M-9321/0	hamartoma, peripheral, gingival, epithelial (T-170._)
M-9320/0	myxofibroma (T-170._)
M-9320/0	myxoma (T-170._)
M-9270/3	sarcoma (T-170._)

Odontogenic cyst

M-------	NOS (SNOMED M-26520)
M-9301/0	calcifying (T-170._)
M-------	dentigerous (SNOMED M-26560)
M-------	eruptive (SNOMED M-26550)
M-------	gingival (SNOMED M-26540)
M-------	primordial (SNOMED M-26530)

Odontogenic tumor

M-9270/1	NOS (T-170._)
M-9300/0	adenomatoid (T-170._)
M-9270/0	benign (T-170._)
M-9340/0	calcifying epithelial (T-170._)
M-9270/3	malignant (T-170._)
M-9312/0	squamous (T-170._)

Odontoma

M-9280/0	NOS (T-170._)
M-9282/0	complex (T-170._)
M-9281/0	compound (T-170._)
M-9290/0	fibroameloblastic (T-170._)

M-9290/3	Odontosarcoma, ameloblastic (T-170._)

T------	Oesophagus (see Esophagus)
T-192.0	Olfactory nerve

Olfactory

M-9522/3	neuroblastoma (T-160._)
M-9523/3	neuroepithelioma (T-160._)
M-9520/3	neurogenic tumor

M-9382/3	Oligo-astrocytoma, mixed (T-191._)
M-9460/3	Oligodendroblastoma (T-191._)
M-9450/3	Oligodendroglioma, NOS (T-191._)
M-9451/3	Oligodendroglioma, anaplastic type (T-191._)

T-191.7	Olive
T-158.8	Omentum

Oncocytic

M-8290/3	adenocarcinoma
M-8290/0	adenoma
M-8290/3	carcinoma

M-8290/0	Oncocytoma
M-------	Oncocytosis *(SNOMED M-73050)*

T-191.0	Operculum

Optic

T-192.0	chiasm
T-192.0	nerve
T-192.0	tract

T-145.9	Oral cavity
T-145.9	Oral mucosa

Orbit

T-190.1	NOS
T-190.1	connective tissue
T-190.1	soft tissue

T-170.0	Orbital bone

M-------	Orbital lymphoma *(SNOMED M-72290)*
M-9071/3	Orchioblastoma (T-186._)

T-194.6	Organ of Zuckerkandl

Organs

T-159.9	digestive, NOS
T-184.9	female genital, NOS
T-187.9	male genital, NOS

T-188.6	Orifice, ureteric
T-188.5	Orifice, urethral, internal

Oropharynx

T-146.9	NOS
T-146.5	junctional region
T-146.6	lateral wall
T-146.7	posterior wall

T-180.1	Os, external
T-180.0	Os, internal

M-9262/0	Ossifying fibroma (T-170._)
M-------	Osteitis deformans *(SNOMED M-74970)*
M-------	Osteitis fibrosa cystica *(SNOMED M-74840)*

M-9180/3	Osteoblastic sarcoma (T-170._)
M-9200/0	Osteoblastoma (T-170._)
M-9210/0	Osteocartilaginous exostosis (T-170._)
M-9210/0	Osteochondroma (T-170._)
M-9210/1	Osteochondromatosis, NOS (T-170._)
M-------	Osteochondromatosis, synovial *(SNOMED M-73670)*
M-9180/3	Osteochondrosarcoma (T-170._)
M-9250/1	Osteoclastoma, NOS (T-170._)
M-9250/3	Osteoclastoma, malignant (T-170._)
M-9262/0	Osteofibroma (T-170._)
M-9182/3	Osteofibrosarcoma (T-170._)

Osteogenic sarcoma

M-9180/3	NOS (T-170._)
M-9190/3	juxtacortical (T-170._)
M-9190/3	periosteal (T-170._)

M-9191/0	Osteoid osteoma, NOS (T-170._)
M-9200/0	Osteoid osteoma, giant (T-170._)

Osteoma

M-9180/0	NOS (T-170._)
M-9191/0	osteoid, NOS (T-170._)
M-9200/0	osteoid, giant (T-170._)

Osteosarcoma

M-9180/3	NOS (T-170._)
M-9181/3	chondroblastic (T-170._)
M-9182/3	fibroblastic (T-170._)
M-9190/3	juxtacortical (T-170._)
M-9190/3	parosteal (T-170._)
M-9183/3	telangiectatic (T-170._)

M-9184/3	Osteosarcoma in Paget's disease of bone (T-170._)

T-174.8	Outer breast
T-173.1	Outer canthus

M-8590/1	Ovarian stromal tumor (T-183.0)

T-183.0	Ovary

M-8290/3	Oxyphilic adenocarcinoma
M-8290/0	Oxyphilic adenoma

- P -

M-9507/0 Pacinian tumor

Paget's disease

M-8541/3	and infiltrating duct carcinoma of breast (T-174._)
M-------	bone *(SNOMED M-74970)*
M-9184/3	bone, osteosarcoma in (T-170._)
M-8540/3	breast (T-174._)
M-8542/3	extramammary *(except Paget's disease of bone)*
M-8540/3	mammary (T-174._)

Palate

T-145.5	NOS
T-145.2	hard
T-145.5	junction of hard and soft
T-145.3	soft, NOS *(excludes Nasopharyngeal surface T-147.3)*
T-147.3	soft, nasopharyngeal surface

T-146.0	Palatine tonsil
T-191.0	Pallium
T-173.6	Palm, skin

Palmar

T-171.2	aponeurosis
T-171.2	fascia
T-173.6	skin

T-173.1	Palpebra

Pancreas

T-157.9	NOS
T-157.1	body
T-157.3	duct
T-157.3	duct, Santorini
T-157.3	duct, Wirsung
T-157.0	head
T-157.4	islands of Langerhans
T-157.4	islets of Langerhans
T-157.2	tail

T-157.3	Pancreatic duct
T-196.2	Pancreatic lymph node

M-9951/1 Panmyelosis, acute (T-169.1)

Papillary

M-8260/0	adenoma, NOS
M-8504/0	adenoma, intracystic
M-------	cystitis *(SNOMED M-76820)*
M-9393/1	ependymoma (T-191._)
M-8052/3	epidermoid carcinoma
M-8405/0	hidradenoma (T-173._)
M-9538/1	meningioma (T-192._)
M-8052/3	squamous cell carcinoma
M-8406/0	syringadenoma (T-173._)
M-8406/0	syringocystadenoma (T-173._)
M-8130/3	transitional cell carcinoma

Papillary adenocarcinoma

M-8260/3	NOS
M-8503/2	non-infiltrating, intraductal
M-8460/3	serous (T-183.0)

Papillary and follicular

M-8340/3	adenocarcinoma (T-193.9)
M-8340/3	carcinoma (T-193.9)
M-8340/3	carcinoma, mixed (T-193.9)

Papillary carcinoma

M-8050/3	NOS
M-8052/3	epidermoid
M-8050/2	in-situ
M-8503/2	non-infiltrating, intraductal
M-8461/3	serous surface (T-183.0)
M-8052/3	squamous cell
M-8130/3	transitional cell

Papillary cystadenocarcinoma

M-8450/3	NOS (T-183.0)
M-8471/3	mucinous (T-183.0)
M-8471/3	pseudomucinous (T-183.0)
M-8460/3	serous (T-183.0)

Papillary cystadenoma

M-8450/0	NOS (T-183.0)
M-8450/1	borderline malignancy (T-183.0)
M-8561/0	lymphomatosum (T-142._)
M-8471/0	mucinous, NOS (T-183.0)
M-8471/1	mucinous, borderline malignancy (T-183.0)
M-8471/0	pseudomucinous, NOS (T-183.0)
M-8471/1	pseudomucinous, borderline malignancy (T-183.0)
M-8460/0	serous, NOS (T-183.0)
M-8460/1	serous, borderline malignancy (T-183.0)

M------- Papilliferous hyperplasia *(SNOMED M-72050)*
M-8450/3 Papillocystic adenocarcinoma

Papilloma

M-8050/0 NOS *(except Papilloma of urinary bladder M-8120/1)*
M------- basal cell *(SNOMED M-72750)*
M------- basosquamous *(SNOMED M-72750)*
M-9390/0 choroid plexus, NOS **(T-191.5)**
M-9390/3 choroid plexus, anaplastic type **(T-191.5)**
M-9390/3 choroid plexus, malignant **(T-191.5)**
M-8503/0 ductal
M-8052/0 dyskeratotic
M------- fibroepithelial *(SNOMED M-76810)*
M-8052/0 hyperkeratotic
M-8504/0 intracystic
M-8503/0 intraductal
M-8053/0 inverted
M-8052/0 keratotic
M-8052/0 parakeratotic
M-8121/0 Schneiderian
M-8461/0 serous surface, NOS **(T-183.0)**
M-8461/1 serous surface, borderline malignancy **(T-183.0)**
M-8052/0 squamous
M-8052/0 squamous cell
M-8120/0 transitional
M-8120/0 transitional cell, NOS
M-8121/1 transitional cell, inverted type
M-8120/1 urinary bladder **(T-188._)**
M-8120/1 urothelial
M-8051/0 verrucous
M-8261/1 villous

Papillomatosis

M-8060/0 NOS
M-8505/0 intraductal, NOS
M-8505/0 intraductal, diffuse
M-8506/0 subareolar duct **(T-174.0)**

M-8263/0 Papillotubular adenoma
M------- Papulosis, lymphomatoid *(SNOMED M-72230)*

T-194.6 Para-aortic body
T-196.2 Para-aortic lymph node
T-196.6 Paracervical lymph node

M-8510/3 Parafollicular cell carcinoma **(T-193.9)**

Paraganglioma

M-8680/1 NOS
M-8691/1 aortic body **(T-194.6)**

Paraganglioma (Cont'd)

M-8692/1 carotid body **(T-194.5)**
M-8700/0 chromaffin
M-8693/1 extra-adrenal, NOS
M-8693/3 extra-adrenal, malignant
M-8690/1 jugular **(T-194.6)**
M-8680/3 malignant
M-8693/1 nonchromaffin, NOS
M-8693/3 nonchromaffin, malignant
M-8682/1 parasympathetic
M-8681/1 sympathetic

T-194.6 Paraganglion

M-9660/3 Paragranuloma, Hodgkin's
M-8052/0 Parakeratotic papilloma

T-196.6 Parametrial lymph node
T-183.4 Parametrium
T-160.9 Paranasal sinus
T-192.9 Parasellar
T-196.1 Parasternal lymph node
T-171.9 Parasympathetic nervous system

M-8682/1 Parasympathetic paraganglioma

T-194.1 Parathyroid gland
T-189.4 Paraurethral gland
T-189.0 Parenchyma, kidney

Parietal

T-170.0 bone
T-191.3 lobe
T-163.0 pleura

M-9190/3 Parosteal osteosarcoma **(T-170._)**

Parotid

T-142.0 NOS
T-142.0 gland
T-142.0 gland duct
T-196.0 lymph node

T-183.3 Parovarian region
T-170.8 Patella
T-196.3 Pectoral lymph node
T-171.4 Pectoralis major muscle
T-191.7 Peduncle, cerebral

Pelvic

T-170.6	bone
T-153.3	colon
T-196.6	lymph node
T-158.8	peritoneum
T-195.3	wall, NOS

T-154.0 Pelvi-rectal junction

Pelvis

T-195.3	NOS
T-171.6	NOS (sarcoma, lipoma)
T-170.6	bone
T-171.6	connective tissue
T-171.6	fibrous tissue
T-171.6	muscle
T-171.6	skeletal muscle
T-171.6	soft tissue
T-195.3	wall, NOS

T-189.1 Pelvis, kidney
T-189.1 Pelvis, renal
T-189.1 Pelvi-ureteric junction

Penis

T-187.4	NOS
T-187.3	body
T-187.3	corpus
T-187.3	corpus cavernosum
T-187.1	foreskin
T-187.2	glans
T-187.1	prepuce
T-187.4	skin

T-158.0 Periadrenal tissue
T-156.2 Periampullary
T-173.5 Perianal skin
T-196.2 Periaortic lymph node

M------- Periapical cemental dysplasia
         (SNOMED M-74870)
M-9012/0 Pericanalicular fibroadenoma (T-174._)

T-164.1 Pericardium
T-158.0 Perinephric tissue

Perineum

T-195.3	NOS
T-173.5	NOS (carcinoma, melanoma, nevus)
T-171.6	NOS (sarcoma, lipoma)
T-171.6	connective tissue

Perineum (Cont'd)

T-171.6	fibrous tissue
T-171.6	muscle
T-171.6	skeletal muscle
T-173.5	skin
T-171.6	soft tissue
T-171.6	subcutaneous tissue

T-143.9 Periodontal tissue

Periosteal

M-9221/0	chondroma (T-170._)
M-8812/0	fibroma (T-170._)
M-8812/3	fibrosarcoma (T-170._)
M-8812/3	sarcoma, NOS (T-170._)
M-9190/3	sarcoma, osteogenic (T-170._)

T-196.2 Peripancreatic lymph node
T-158.0 Peripancreatic tissue
T-171.9 Peripheral nerve, NOS

M------- Peripheral odontogenic fibroma
         (SNOMED M-76850)
M-9321/0 Peripheral odontogenic gingival epithelial
         hamartoma (T-170._)

T-195.3 Perirectal region, NOS
T-158.0 Perirenal tissue
T-158.9 Peritoneal cavity

Peritoneum

T-158.9	NOS
T-158.9	cavity
T-158.8	cul de sac
T-158.8	mesentery
T-158.8	mesoappendix
T-158.8	mesocolon
T-158.8	omentum
T-158.8	pelvic
T-158.8	pouch, Douglas
T-158.8	pouch, rectouterine

M------- Peutz-Jeghers polyp *(SNOMED M-75630)*

T-170.8 Phalanx of foot
T-170.5 Phalanx of hand

Pharyngeal

T-147.3	fornix
T-147.1	tonsil
T-149.0	wall, NOS

Pharynx
T-149.0   NOS
T-149.0   wall, NOS
T-149.0   wall, lateral, NOS
T-149.0   wall, posterior, NOS

M-8700/3 Pheochromoblastoma (T-194.0)
M-8700/0 Pheochromocytoma, NOS (T-194.0)
M-8700/3 Pheochromocytoma, malignant (T-194.0)

Pia mater
T-192.1   NOS
T-192.1   cranial
T-192.3   spinal

M-8640/0 Pick's tubular adenoma

Pigmented
M-8090/3   basal cell carcinoma (T-173._)
M-8720/0   nevus, NOS (T-173._)
M-8761/1   nevus, giant (T-173._)
M-8761/3   nevus, giant, malignant melanoma in
            (T-173._)
M-------   villonodular synovitis (SNOMED M-47830)

M-------   Pilar cyst (SNOMED M-33470)

T-146.2   Pillar, faucial
T-146.2   Pillar, tonsillar

M-9421/3 Pilocytic astrocytoma (T-191._)
M-9421/3 Piloid astrocytoma (T-191._)
M-8110/0 Pilomatrixoma (T-173._)

T-194.4   Pineal gland

M-9360/1 Pinealoma (T-194.4)
M-9362/3 Pineoblastoma (T-194.4)
M-9361/1 Pineocytoma (T-194.4)

T-173.2   Pinna

Pituitary
T-194.3   NOS
T-194.3   fossa
T-194.3   gland

T-181.9   Placenta

Plantar
T-171.3   aponeurosis
T-171.3   fascia
T-173.7   skin

Plasma cell
M-------   granuloma (SNOMED M-43060)
M-9830/3 leukemia (T-169._)
M-9730/3 myeloma
M-------   pseudotumor (SNOMED M-43060)
M-9731/3 sarcoma

Plasma cell tumor
M-9731/1   NOS
M-9731/0   benign
M-9731/3   malignant

M-9830/3 Plasmacytic leukemia (T-169._)
M-9730/3 Plasmacytic myeloma

Plasmacytoma
M-9731/1   NOS
M-9731/0   benign
M-9731/1   solitary

Pleomorphic
M-8940/0   adenoma
M-8940/3   adenoma, carcinoma in
M-8022/3   carcinoma
M-8802/3   cell sarcoma
M-8854/3   liposarcoma
M-8901/3   rhabdomyosarcoma

Pleomorphic cell type
M-9641/3   malignant lymphoma, histiocytic
M-9641/3   reticulosarcoma
M-9641/3   reticulum cell sarcoma

Pleura
T-163.9   NOS
T-163.0   parietal
T-163.1   visceral

Plexiform
M-9131/0   hemangioma
M-9550/0   neurofibroma
M-9550/0   neuroma

Plexus

T-171.2	brachial
T-171.0	cervical
T-191.5	choroid
T-171.6	lumbosacral
T-171.6	sacral

T-194.8   Pluriglandular

M-8981/3   Pneumoblastoma (T-162._)

T-191.1   Pole, frontal
T-191.4   Pole, occipital

Polycythemia

M-9950/1	rubra vera (T-169._)
M-------	secondary (SNOMED M-77720)
M-9950/1	vera (T-169._)

M-9072/3   Polyembryoma
M-9072/3   Polyembryonal type embryonal carcinoma
M-8034/3   Polygonal cell carcinoma

Polyp

M-------	NOS (SNOMED M-76800)
M-8210/0	adenomatous, NOS
M-8210/3	adenomatous, adenocarcinoma in
M-8210/3	adenomatous, carcinoma in
M-------	fibroepithelial (SNOMED M-76810)
M-------	fibrous (SNOMED M-76810)
M-------	hyperplastic (SNOMED M-72040)
M-------	inflammatory (SNOMED M-76820)
M-------	juvenile (SNOMED M-75640)
M-------	lymphoid, NOS (SNOMED M-76880)
M-------	lymphoid, benign (SNOMED M-76880)
M-------	metaplastic (SNOMED M-72040)
M-------	Peutz-Jeghers (SNOMED M-75630)

M-8210/0   Polypoid adenoma
M-8210/3   Polypoid adenoma, adenocarcinoma in

Polyposis

M-8220/0	adenomatous, coli (T-153._)
M-8220/3	adenomatous, coli, adenocarcinoma in (T-153._)
M-8220/0	coli, familial (T-153._)
M-8221/0	multiple

M-8221/0   Polyps, adenomatous, multiple
M-9071/3   Polyvesicular vitelline tumor

T-191.7   Pons

M-____/_(3) Poorly differentiated (see Grading code, page 20)

T-196.5   Popliteal lymph node

Popliteal space

T-195.5	NOS
T-173.7	NOS (carcinoma, melanoma, nevus)
T-171.3	NOS (sarcoma, lipoma)
T-171.3	adipose tissue
T-171.3	connective tissue
T-171.3	fatty tissue
T-171.3	fibrous tissue
T-173.7	skin
T-171.3	soft tissue
T-171.3	subcutaneous tissue
T-171.3	tendon
T-171.3	tendon sheath

M-8402/0   Poroma, eccrine (T-173._)

T-196.2   Porta-hepatis lymph node
T-196.2   Portal lymph node

M-------   Portwine nevus (SNOMED M-75540)

T-148.0   Postcricoid region

Posterior

T-191.9	cranial fossa
T-147.3	margin of nasal septum
T-164.3	mediastinum
T-161.1	surface of epiglottis
T-141.0	third of tongue
T-141.0	tongue, NOS

Posterior wall

T-148.3	hypopharynx
T-146.7	mesopharynx
T-147.1	nasopharynx
T-146.7	oropharynx
T-149.0	pharynx, NOS
T-151.8	stomach, NOS (not classifiable to T-151.0 to T-151.4)
T-188.4	urinary bladder

Pouch

T-158.8	Douglas's
T-194.3	Rathke's
T-158.8	rectouterine

T-196.0   Preauricular lymph node

M-8741/2 Precancerous melanosis, NOS (T-173._)
M-8741/3 Precancerous melanosis, malignant melanoma
          in (T-173._)
M------- Pregnancy luteoma (SNOMED M-79680)

T-196.0   Prelaryngeal lymph node
T-187.1   Prepuce
T-151.1   Prepylorus
T-195.3   Presacral region, NOS
T-196.6   Presymphysial lymph node
T-196.0   Pretracheal lymph node

M-____/3 Primary site, malignant (see Behavior code,
          page 20)

T-199.9   Primary site unknown

M-9443/3 Primitive polar spongioblastoma (T-191._)
M------- Primordial cyst (SNOMED M-26530)
M-9363/0 Progonoma, melanotic
M-9000/1 Proliferating Brenner tumor (T-183.0)
M-9825/3 Prolymphocytic leukemia (T-169._)
M-9631/3 Prolymphocytic lymphosarcoma

T-185.9   Prostate, NOS
T-185.9   Prostate gland
T-189.3   Prostatic utricle

M-9410/3 Protoplasmic astrocytoma (T-191._)

T-150.3   Proximal third of esophagus

M-9533/0 Psammomatous meningioma (T-192._)
M------- Pseudoepitheliomatous hyperplasia
          (SNOMED M-72090)
M-8075/3 Pseudoglandular squamous cell carcinoma
M------- Pseudolymphoma (SNOMED M-72290)

Pseudomucinous
M-8470/3 adenocarcinoma (T-183.0)
M-8470/3 cystadenocarcinoma, NOS (T-183.0)
M-8471/3 cystadenocarcinoma, papillary (T-183.0)

Pseudomucinous cystadenoma
M-8470/0 NOS (T-183.0)
M-8470/1 borderline malignancy (T-183.0)
M-8471/0 papillary, NOS (T-183.0)
M-8471/1 papillary, borderline malignancy (T-183.0)

M-8480/6 Pseudomyxoma peritonei (T-158.9)
M------- Pseudopolyp, NOS (SNOMED M-76820)
M------- Pseudosarcoma (SNOMED M-76190)

Pseudosarcomatous
M-8033/3 carcinoma
M------- fasciitis (SNOMED M-76130)
M------- fibromatosis (SNOMED M-76130)

Pseudotumor
M------- NOS (SNOMED M-03090)
M------- inflammatory (SNOMED M-76820)
M------- plasma cell (SNOMED M-43060)

T-171.5   Psoas muscle

Pterygoid fossa
T-171.0   NOS
T-171.0   connective tissue
T-171.0   fibrous tissue
T-171.0   soft tissue

T-170.6   Pubic bone
T-184.4   Pudendum

Pulmonary
T-162.9   NOS
T-196.1   lymph node, NOS
T-196.1   lymph node, hilar

M-8250/1 Pulmonary adenomatosis (T-162._)
M-8331/3 Pure follicle type, follicular adenocarcinoma
          (T-193.9)
M-8331/3 Pure follicle type, follicular carcinoma
          (T-193.9)

T-191.0   Putamen

Pyloric
T-151.2   antrum
T-151.1   canal
T-196.2   lymph node

T-151.1   Pylorus

M------- Pyogenic granuloma (SNOMED M-44440)

T-191.7   Pyramid
T-148.1   Pyriform fossa
T-148.1   Pyriform sinus

- Q -

T-171.3   Quadriceps femoris muscle

M-8080/2 Queyrat's erythroplasia (T-187.__)

- R -

M-9123/0 Racemose hemangioma

T-171.2   Radial artery
T-171.2   Radial nerve

M-------   Radicular cyst *(SNOMED M-43800)*

T-170.4   Radius
T-194.3   Rathke's pouch

M-9350/1 Rathke's pouch tumor (T-194.3)
M-9540/1 Recklinghausen's disease *(except of Bone)*
M-------   Recklinghausen's disease of bone
            (SNOMED M-74840)

T-154.1   Rectal ampulla

Rectosigmoid
T-154.0   NOS
T-154.0   colon
T-154.0   junction

T-158.8   Rectouterine pouch
T-195.3   Rectovaginal septum
T-195.3   Rectovesical septum
T-154.1   Rectum, NOS
T-154.0   Rectum and colon
T-171.5   Rectus abdominis muscle

Renal
T-189.0   NOS
T-171.5   artery
T-189.1   calyces
T-189.1   calyx
T-189.1   pelvis

M-8312/3 Renal cell adenocarcinoma (T-189.0)
M-8312/3 Renal cell carcinoma (T-189.0)

M-8361/1 Reninoma (T-189.0)
M-8041/3 Reserve cell carcinoma

T-165.9   Respiratory tract, NOS
T-165.0   Respiratory tract, upper

M-------   Rest, embryonal, NOS *(SNOMED M-26300)*
M-------   Rest, Walthard's *(SNOMED M-26350)*

T-186.0   Retained testis *(site of neoplasm)*
T-169.3   Reticuloendothelial system, NOS

Reticuloendotheliosis
M-9722/3   acute infantile
M-9940/3   leukemic
M-9720/3   malignant
M-9722/3   non-lipid

M-------   Reticulohistiocytic granuloma
            (SNOMED M-77880)
M-------   Reticulohistiocytoma *(SNOMED M-77880)*

Reticulolymphosarcoma
M-9613/3   NOS
M-9613/3   diffuse
M-9691/3   follicular
M-9691/3   nodular

Reticulosarcoma
M-9640/3   NOS
M-9642/3   nodular
M-9641/3   pleomorphic cell type

Reticulosis
M-9722/3   acute, infancy
M-9721/3   histiocytic medullary
M-9720/3   malignant

M-9640/3 Reticulum cell sarcoma, NOS
M-9641/3 Reticulum cell sarcoma, pleomorphic cell type

T-190.5   Retina

M-9363/0 Retinal anlage tumor

Retinoblastoma
M-9510/3   NOS (T-190.5)
M-9511/3   differentiated type (T-190.5)
M-9512/3   undifferentiated type (T-190.5)

T-190.1   Retrobulbar tissue
T-158.0   Retrocecal tissue

Retromolar
T-145.6   area
T-145.6   triangle
T-145.6   trigone

T-196.2   Retroperitoneal lymph node
T-158.0   Retroperitoneal tissue
T-158.0   Retroperitoneum
T-196.0   Retropharyngeal lymph node
T-149.0   Retropharynx

Rhabdomyoma
M-8900/0   NOS
M-8904/0   adult
M-8903/0   fetal
M-8904/0   glycogenic

Rhabdomyosarcoma
M-8900/3   NOS
M-8920/3   alveolar
M-8910/3   embryonal
M-8902/3   mixed type
M-8901/3   pleomorphic

M-8900/3   Rhabdosarcoma

T-191.0   Rhinencephalon
T-170.3   Rib
T-153.6   Right colon

M-8090/3   Rodent ulcer (T-173._)

T-145.5   Roof of mouth
T-147.0   Roof of nasopharynx
T-141.0   Root of tongue
T-147.2   Rosenmüller's fossa
T-196.5   Rosenmüller's lymph node

Round cell
M-8041/3   carcinoma
M-8853/3   liposarcoma
M-8803/3   sarcoma

T-183.5   Round ligament

M-------   Rugal hypertrophy, giant
              (SNOMED M-71330)

- S -

T-190.7   Sac, lacrimal

Sacral
T-192.2   cord
T-196.6   lymph node
T-171.6   nerve
T-171.6   plexus

Sacrococcygeal region
T-195.3   NOS
T-173.5   NOS (carcinoma, melanoma, nevus)
T-171.6   NOS (sarcoma, lipoma)
T-171.6   adipose tissue
T-171.6   connective tissue
T-171.6   fatty tissue
T-171.6   fibrous tissue
T-171.6   muscle
T-171.6   skeletal muscle
T-173.5   skin
T-171.6   soft tissue
T-171.6   subcutaneous tissue

T-170.6   Sacrum

Salivary gland
T-142.9   NOS *(excludes Minor salivary gland; see Introduction page xviii and note under T-142)*
T-142.9   major, NOS
T-145.9   minor, NOS *(see Introduction page xviii and note under T-142)*

M-8940/0   Salivary gland type mixed tumor, NOS
M-8940/3   Salivary gland type mixed tumor, malignant
M-------   Salpingitis isthmica nodosa
              (SNOMED M-74200)

T-157.3   Santorini's duct

M-------   Sarcoid granuloma *(SNOMED M-44210)*

Sarcoma
M-8800/3   NOS
M-9581/3   alveolar soft part
M-9330/3   ameloblastic (T-170._)
M-8910/3   botryoid
M-8910/3   botryoides
M-9480/3   cerebellar, NOS (T-191.6)
M-9471/3   circumscribed arachnoidal cerebellar
              (T-191.6)

Sarcoma (Cont'd)

M-9044/3   clear cell of tendons and aponeuroses (T-171._)

M-8991/3   embryonal

M-8930/3   endometrial, NOS (T-182.0)

M-8930/3   endometrial stromal (T-182.0)

M-9260/3   endothelial, bone (T-170._)

M-8804/3   epithelioid cell

M-9260/3   Ewing's (T-170._)

M-9632/3   germinoblastic, NOS

M-9632/3   germinoblastic, diffuse

M-9697/3   germinoblastic, follicular

M-8802/3   giant cell

M-9250/3   giant cell, bone (T-170._)

M-8710/3   glomoid

M-9930/3   granulocytic

M-9130/3   hemangioendothelial

M-9662/3   Hodgkin's

M-9612/3   immunoblastic

M-9140/3   Kaposi's

M-9124/3   Kupffer cell (T-155.0)

M-9530/3   leptomeningeal (T-192._)

M-9170/3   lymphangioendothelial

M-9740/3   mast cell

M-9530/3   meningeal (T-192._)

M-9530/3   meningothelial (T-192._)

M-8990/3   mesenchymal, mixed

M-9050/3   mesothelial

M-9481/3   monstrocellular (T-191._)

M-9140/3   multiple hemorrhagic

M-9930/3   myeloid

M-9540/3   neurogenic

M-9270/3   odontogenic (T-170._)

M-9180/3   osteoblastic (T-170._)

M-9180/3   osteogenic, NOS (T-170._)

M-9190/3   osteogenic, juxtacortical (T-170._)

M-9190/3   osteogenic, periosteal (T-170._)

M-8812/3   periosteal, NOS (T-170._)

M-9731/3   plasma cell

M-8802/3   pleomorphic cell

M-9640/3   reticulum cell, NOS

M-9641/3   reticulum cell, pleomorphic cell type

M-8803/3   round cell

M-8803/3   small cell

M-8801/3   spindle cell

M-8930/3   stromal, NOS

M-8930/3   stromal, endometrial (T-182.0)

M-9040/3   synovial, NOS

M-9043/3   synovial, biphasic type

M-9042/3   synovial, epithelioid cell type

M-9041/3   synovial, spindle cell type

M-8800/9   Sarcomatosis, NOS

M-9539/3   Sarcomatosis, meningeal (T-192._)

T-196.0   Scalene lymph node

Scalp

T-173.4   NOS

T-173.4   NOS (carcinoma, melanoma, nevus)

T-171.0   NOS (sarcoma, lipoma)

T-171.0   adipose tissue

T-171.0   connective tissue

T-171.0   fatty tissue

T-171.0   fibrous tissue

T-171.0   muscle

T-171.0   skeletal muscle

T-173.4   skin

T-171.0   soft tissue

T-171.0   subcutaneous tissue

T-170.4   Scapula

Scapular region

T-195.1   NOS

T-173.5   NOS (carcinoma, melanoma, nevus)

T-171.4   NOS (sarcoma, lipoma)

T-171.4   adipose tissue

T-171.4   connective tissue

T-171.4   fatty tissue

T-171.4   fibrous tissue

T-173.5   skin

T-171.4   soft tissue

T-171.4   subcutaneous tissue

M-------   Scar, hyperplastic *(SNOMED M-49730)*

M-8121/3   Schneiderian carcinoma

M-8121/0   Schneiderian papilloma

M-9560/0   Schwannoma, NOS

M-9560/3   Schwannoma, malignant

T-171.3   Sciatic nerve

M-8141/3   Scirrhous adenocarcinoma

M-8141/3   Scirrhous carcinoma

T-190.0   Sclera

Sclerosing

M-8350/3   adenocarcinoma, nonencapsulated (T-193.9)

M-------   adenosis *(SNOMED M-74220)*

M-8350/3   carcinoma, nonencapsulated (T-193.9)

M-8832/0   hemangioma (T-173._)

M-8350/3   tumor, nonencapsulated (T-193.9)

T-186.9 Scrotal testis
T-187.7 Scrotum, NOS
T-187.7 Scrotum, skin

Sebaceous
M-8410/3 adenocarcinoma (T-173._)
M-8410/0 adenoma (T-173._)
M-8410/3 carcinoma (T-173._)
M------- cyst (SNOMED M-33430)

M------- Seborrheic keratosis (SNOMED M-72750)
M------- Seborrheic verruca (SNOMED M-72750)
M-____/6 Secondary site (see Behavior code, page 20)

Secondary
M-8010/6 carcinoma
M-8000/6 neoplasm
M------- polycythemia (SNOMED M-77720)
M-8000/6 tumor

M-8502/3 Secretory carcinoma of the breast (T-174._)

T-194.3 Sella turcica
T-170.7 Semilunar cartilage
T-187.8 Seminal vesicle

Seminoma
M-9061/3 NOS (T-186._)
M-9062/3 anaplastic type (T-186._)
M-9063/3 spermatocytic (T-186._)

M------- Senile keratosis (SNOMED M-72850)

Septum
T-160.0 nasal, NOS (excludes Posterior margin of nasal septum T-147.3)
T-147.3 nasal, posterior margin
T-195.3 rectovaginal
T-195.3 rectovesical
T-184.9 urethrovaginal
T-184.9 vesicovaginal

Serous
M-8441/3 adenocarcinoma, NOS
M-8460/3 adenocarcinoma, papillary (T-183.0)
M-9014/0 adenofibroma (T-183.0)
M-8441/3 cystadenocarcinoma, NOS (T-183.0)
M-8460/3 cystadenocarcinoma, papillary (T-183.0)
M-9014/0 cystadenofibroma (T-183.0)
M-8441/0 cystoma (T-183.0)

Serous cystadenoma
M-8441/0 NOS (T-183.0)
M-8441/1 borderline malignancy (T-183.0)
M-8460/0 papillary, NOS (T-183.0)
M-8460/1 papillary, borderline malignancy (T-183.0)

Serous surface
M-8461/3 carcinoma, papillary (T-183.0)
M-8461/0 papilloma, NOS (T-183.0)
M-8461/1 papilloma, borderline malignancy (T-183.0)

Sertoli cell
M-8640/0 adenoma
M-8640/3 carcinoma (T-186._)
M-8640/0 tumor, NOS
M-8641/0 tumor with lipid storage

M-8631/0 Sertoli-Leydig cell tumor
M-8590/1 Sex cord tumor
M-8590/1 Sex cord-stromal tumor
M-9701/3 Sezary's disease
M-9701/3 Sezary's syndrome

Shoulder
T-195.4 NOS
T-173.6 NOS (carcinoma, melanoma, nevus)
T-171.2 NOS (sarcoma, lipoma)
T-171.2 adipose tissue
T-170.4 bone
T-171.2 connective tissue
T-171.2 fatty tissue
T-171.2 fibrous tissue
T-170.4 girdle
T-170.4 joint
T-171.2 muscle
T-171.2 skeletal muscle
T-173.6 skin
T-171.2 soft tissue
T-171.2 subcutaneous tissue

Sigmoid
T-153.3 NOS
T-153.3 colon
T-153.3 flexure of colon

Signet ring cell
M-8490/3 adenocarcinoma
M-8490/3 carcinoma
M-8490/6 carcinoma, metastatic

Sinus

T-160.9	accessory, NOS
T-160.9	accessory, nasal
T-160.3	ethmoid
T-160.4	frontal
T-160.2	maxillary
T-160.9	paranasal
T-148.1	pyriform
T-160.5	sphenoid

M------- Sinus histiocytosis with massive
lymphadenopathy *(SNOMED M-77940)*

Site

T-191.9	intracranial
T-195.2	intra-abdominal, NOS
T-195.1	intrathoracic, NOS
T-199.9	primary, unknown

T-170.9 Skeletal bone

Skeletal muscle

T-171.9	NOS
T-171.5	abdominal wall
T-171.2	arm
T-171.7	back
T-171.6	buttock
T-171.3	calf
T-171.4	chest wall
T-171.0	face
T-171.2	finger
T-171.7	flank
T-171.3	foot
T-171.2	forearm
T-171.2	hand
T-171.0	head
T-171.3	leg
T-171.0	neck
T-171.6	perineum
T-171.6	sacrococcygeal region
T-171.0	scalp
T-171.2	shoulder
T-171.3	thigh
T-171.4	thoracic wall
T-171.2	thumb
T-171.3	toe
T-171.7	trunk

Skin

T-173.9 NOS *(excludes Skin of labia majora
T-184.1, Skin of vulva T-184.4, Skin of
penis T-187.4 and Skin of Scrotum
T-187.7)*

Skin (Cont'd)

T-173.5	abdomen
T-173.5	abdominal wall
T-173.3	ala nasi
T-173.7	ankle
T-173.6	antecubital space
T-173.5	anus
T-173.6	arm
T-173.2	auditory canal, NOS
T-173.2	auditory canal, external
T-173.2	auditory meatus, external
T-173.2	auricle
T-173.2	auricular canal, NOS
T-173.2	auricular canal, external
T-173.5	axilla
T-173.5	back
T-173.5	breast
T-173.3	brow
T-173.5	buttock
T-173.7	calf
T-173.1	canthus, NOS
T-173.1	canthus, inner
T-173.1	canthus, outer
T-173.4	cervical region
T-173.3	cheek
T-173.5	chest
T-173.5	chest wall
T-173.3	chin
T-173.3	columnella
T-173.2	concha
T-173.2	ear
T-173.2	ear canal
T-173.2	ear, external
T-173.2	ear lobule
T-173.2	earlobe
T-173.6	elbow
T-173.3	eyebrow
T-173.1	eyelid
T-173.3	face
T-173.6	finger
T-173.5	flank
T-173.7	foot
T-173.6	forearm
T-173.3	forehead
T-173.5	gluteal region
T-173.5	groin
T-173.6	hand
T-173.4	head, NOS
T-173.7	heel
T-173.2	helix
T-173.7	hip
T-173.5	infraclavicular region

Skin (Cont'd)

T-173.5	inguinal region
T-173.1	inner canthus
T-173.3	jaw
T-173.7	knee
T-184.1	labia majora
T-173.7	leg
T-173.1	lid, NOS
T-173.1	lid, lower
T-173.1	lid, upper
T-173.7	limb, lower
T-173.6	limb, upper
T-173.0	lip, NOS
T-173.0	lip, lower
T-173.0	lip, upper
T-173.4	neck
T-173.3	nose
T-173.1	outer canthus
T-173.6	palm
T-173.6	palmar
T-173.1	palpebra
T-187.4	penis
T-173.5	perianal
T-173.5	perineum
T-173.2	pinna
T-173.7	plantar
T-173.7	popliteal space
T-173.5	sacrococcygeal region
T-173.4	scalp
T-173.5	scapular region
T-187.7	scrotum
T-173.6	shoulder
T-173.7	sole, foot
T-173.4	supraclavicular region
T-173.3	temple
T-173.7	thigh
T-173.5	thoracic wall
T-173.5	thorax
T-173.6	thumb
T-173.7	toe
T-173.2	tragus
T-173.5	trunk
T-173.5	umbilicus
T-184.4	vulva
T-173.6	wrist

Skin appendage

M-8390/0	adenoma (T-173._)
M-8390/3	carcinoma (T-173._)
M-8390/0	tumor (T-173._)

T-170.0	Skull, NOS
T-170.0	Skull, bone
T-152.9	Small bowel

Small cell carcinoma

M-8041/3	NOS
M-8073/3	epidermoid, non-keratinizing type
M-8043/3	fusiform cell type
M-8073/3	squamous cell, non-keratinizing type

M-8803/3	Small cell sarcoma
M-8002/3	Small cell type, malignant tumor

T-152.9	Small intestine
T-143.9	Socket, tooth

M-8851/0	Soft fibroma

Soft palate

T-145.3	NOS (excludes Nasopharyngeal surface T-147.3)
T-147.3	nasopharyngeal surface
T-145.5	and hard palate, junction

M-9581/3	Soft part sarcoma, alveolar

Soft tissue

T-171.9	NOS
T-171.5	abdomen
T-171.5	abdominal wall
T-171.3	ankle
T-171.2	antecubital space
T-171.2	arm
T-171.4	axilla
T-171.7	back
T-171.6	buttock
T-171.3	calf
T-171.0	cervical region
T-171.0	cheek
T-171.4	chest
T-171.4	chest wall
T-171.0	chin
T-171.2	elbow
T-171.0	face
T-171.2	finger
T-171.7	flank
T-171.3	foot
T-171.2	forearm
T-171.0	forehead
T-171.6	gluteal region
T-171.6	groin

Soft tissue (Cont'd)

T-171.2	hand
T-171.0	head
T-171.3	heel
T-171.3	hip
T-171.4	infraclavicular region
T-171.6	inguinal region
T-171.3	knee
T-171.3	leg
T-171.0	neck
T-190.1	orbit
T-171.6	perineum
T-171.3	popliteal space
T-171.0	pterygoid fossa, NOS
T-171.6	sacrococcygeal region
T-171.0	scalp
T-171.4	scapular region
T-171.2	shoulder
T-171.0	supraclavicular region
T-171.0	temple
T-171.3	thigh
T-171.4	thoracic wall
T-171.2	thumb
T-171.3	toe
T-171.7	trunk
T-171.5	umbilicus
T-171.2	wrist

M-8800/0	Soft tissue tumor, benign
M-8800/3	Soft tissue tumor, malignant

T-173.7	Sole of foot

Solid

M-8230/3	carcinoma, NOS
M-8511/3	carcinoma with amyloid stroma (T-193.9)
M-9080/1	teratoma

Solitary

M-------	cyst (SNOMED M-33404)
M-9731/1	myeloma
M-9731/1	plasmacytoma

T-187.6	Spermatic cord

M-9063/3	Spermatocytic seminoma (T-186._)
M-9063/3	Spermatocytoma (T-186._)

T-170.0	Sphenoid bone
T-160.5	Sphenoid sinus

M-8035/3	Spheroidal cell carcinoma

T-154.2	Sphincter, anal
T-156.1	Sphincter of Oddi

Spider

M-------	angioma (SNOMED M-76330)
M-------	nevus (SNOMED M-76330)
M-------	vascular (SNOMED M-76330)

Spinal

T-192.0	accessory nerve
T-192.3	arachnoid
T-170.2	column
T-192.2	cord
T-192.3	dura mater
T-192.3	meninges
T-171.9	nerve, NOS
T-192.3	pia mater

M-8775/3	Spindle cell and epithelioid cell melanoma, mixed
M-8770/0	Spindle cell and epithelioid cell nevus (T-173._)
M-8030/3	Spindle cell and giant cell carcinoma

Spindle cell

M-8032/3	carcinoma
M-8030/3	carcinoma and giant cell carcinoma
M-8857/0	lipoma
M-8770/0	nevus (T-173._)
M-8770/0	nevus and epithelioid cell nevus (T-173._)
M-8801/3	sarcoma

Spindle cell melanoma

M-8772/3	NOS
M-8775/3	and epithelioid cell melanoma, mixed
M-8773/3	type A (T-190.0)
M-8774/3	type B (T-190.0)

Spindle cell type

M-8074/3	epidermoid carcinoma
M-8004/3	malignant tumor
M-8074/3	squamous cell carcinoma
M-9041/3	synovial sarcoma
M-8122/3	transitional cell carcinoma

T-170.2	Spine

M-8070/3	Spinous cell carcinoma
M-8403/0	Spiradenoma, NOS (T-173._)
M-8403/0	Spiradenoma, eccrine (T-173._)

T-169.2 Spleen

Splenic
T-153.7 flexure of colon
T-196.2 lymph node, NOS
T-196.2 lymph node, hilar

Spongioblastoma
M-9422/3 NOS (T-191._)
M-9440/3 multiforme (T-191._)
M-9423/3 polare (T-191._)
M-9443/3 primitive polar (T-191._)

M-9504/3 Spongioneuroblastoma

M------- Spongy nevus, mucosa (SNOMED M-75710)

T-180.8 Squamocolumnar junction, cervix

Squamous
M-8070/3 carcinoma
M------- keratosis, benign (SNOMED M-72760)
M------- metaplasia (SNOMED M-73220)
M-9312/0 odontogenic tumor (T-170._)
M-8052/0 papilloma

Squamous cell carcinoma
M-8070/3 NOS
M-8075/3 adenoid
M-8560/3 and adenocarcinoma, mixed
M-8070/2 in-situ, NOS
M-8076/2 in-situ with questionable stromal invasion (T-180._)
M-8081/2 intraepidermal, Bowen's type (T-173._)
M-8070/2 intraepithelial
M-8071/3 keratinizing type, NOS
M-8071/3 large cell, keratinizing type
M-8072/3 large cell, non-keratinizing type
M-8070/6 metastatic, NOS
M-8076/3 micro-invasive (T-180._)
M-8072/3 non-keratinizing type, NOS
M-8052/3 papillary
M-8075/3 pseudoglandular
M-8073/3 small cell, non-keratinizing type
M-8074/3 spindle cell type
M-8051/3 verrucous

M-8094/3 Squamous-basal cell carcinoma, mixed (T-173._)
M-8070/3 Squamous cell epithelioma
M-8052/0 Squamous cell papilloma
M------- Steatocystoma multiplex (SNOMED M-33450)

Stem cell
M-9801/3 leukemia (T-169._)
M-9601/3 lymphoma
M-9601/3 type, malignant lymphoma

T-142.0 Stensen's duct
T-171.0 Sternocleidomastoid muscle
T-170.3 Sternocostal joint
T-170.3 Sternum

Stomach
T-151.9 NOS
T-151.8 anterior wall, NOS (not classifiable to T-151.0 to T-151.4)
T-151.2 antrum
T-151.2 antrum, gastric
T-151.2 antrum, pyloric
T-151.4 body
T-151.0 cardia, NOS
T-151.0 cardia, gastric
T-151.0 cardio-esophageal junction
T-151.4 corpus
T-151.4 corpus, gastric
T-151.0 esophagogastric junction
T-151.3 fundus
T-151.3 fundus, gastric
T-151.0 gastroesophageal junction
T-151.6 greater curvature, NOS (not classifiable to T-151.0 to T-151.4)
T-151.5 lesser curvature, NOS (not classifiable to T-151.1 to T-151.4)
T-151.8 posterior wall, NOS (not classifiable to T-151.0 to T-151.4)
T-151.1 prepylorus
T-151.2 pyloric antrum
T-151.1 pyloric canal
T-151.1 pylorus

M------- Strawberry nevus (SNOMED M-75540)

T-182.0 Stroma, endometrial

Stromal
M-8931/1 endometriosis (T-182.0)
M------- hyperplasia (SNOMED M-72430)
M-8931/1 myosis, NOS (T-182.0)
M-8931/1 myosis, endolymphatic (T-182.0)
M-8930/3 sarcoma, NOS
M-8930/3 sarcoma, endometrial (T-182.0)

Stromal tumor
M-8590/1 gonadal
M-8590/1 ovarian (T-183.0)
M-8590/1 testicular (T-186._)

M-8931/1 Stromatosis, endometrial (T-182.0)

Struma
M-9090/0 ovarii, NOS (T-183.0)
M-9090/3 ovarii, malignant (T-183.0)
M-8332/3 Wuchernde, Langhans (T-193.9)
M-9091/1 ovarii and carcinoid (T-183.0)

M-9091/1 Strumal carcinoid (T-183.0)

T-180.8 Stump, cervical

M-8506/0 Subareolar duct papillomatosis (T-174.0)

T-171.4 Subclavian artery
T-196.3 Subclavicular lymph node

Subcutaneous tissue
T-171.9 NOS
T-171.5 abdomen
T-171.5 abdominal wall
T-171.3 ankle
T-171.2 antecubital space
T-171.2 arm
T-171.4 axilla
T-171.7 back
T-171.6 buttock
T-171.3 calf
T-171.0 cervical region
T-171.0 cheek
T-171.4 chest
T-171.4 chest wall
T-171.0 chin
T-171.2 elbow
T-171.0 face
T-171.2 finger
T-171.7 flank
T-171.3 foot
T-171.2 forearm
T-171.0 forehead
T-171.6 gluteal region
T-171.6 groin
T-171.2 hand
T-171.0 head
T-171.3 heel
T-171.3 hip
T-171.4 infraclavicular region
T-171.6 inguinal region
T-171.3 knee
T-171.3 leg
T-171.0 neck

Subcutaneous (Cont'd)
T-171.6 perineum
T-171.3 popliteal space
T-171.6 sacrococcygeal region
T-171.0 scalp
T-171.4 scapular region
T-171.2 shoulder
T-171.0 supraclavicular region
T-171.0 temple
T-171.3 thigh
T-171.4 thoracic wall
T-171.4 thorax
T-171.2 thumb
T-171.3 toe
T-171.7 trunk
T-171.5 umbilicus
T-171.2 wrist

Subependymal
M-9383/1 astrocytoma, NOS (T-191._)
M-9384/1 astrocytoma, giant cell (T-191._)
M-9383/1 glioma (T-191._)

M-9383/1 Subependymoma (T-191._)
M-8832/0 Subepidermal nodular fibrosis (T-173._)

T-161.2 Subglottis
T-196.5 Subinguinal lymph node

Sublingual
T-142.2 gland
T-142.2 gland duct
T-196.0 lymph node

T-142.1 Submandibular gland
T-196.0 Submandibular lymph node

Submaxillary
T-142.1 gland
T-142.1 gland duct
T-196.0 lymph node

T-196.0 Submental lymph node
T-196.3 Subscapular lymph node

Sulcus
T-145.1 alveolar
T-145.1 buccal
T-145.1 labial

M-8143/3 Superficial spreading adenocarcinoma
M-8743/3 Superficial spreading melanoma

T-196.2 Superior mesenteric lymph node
T-171.4 Superior vena cava
T-147.0 Superior wall of nasopharynx
T-196.0 Supraclavicular lymph node

Supraclavicular region
T-195.0 NOS
T-173.4 NOS (carcinoma, melanoma, nevus)
T-171.0 NOS (sarcoma, lipoma)
T-171.0 adipose tissue
T-171.0 connective tissue
T-171.0 fatty tissue
T-171.0 fibrous tissue
T-196.0 lymph node
T-173.4 skin
T-171.0 soft tissue
T-171.0 subcutaneous tissue

T-161.1 Supraglottis
T-194.0 Suprarenal gland
T-191.9 Suprasellar

Sweat gland
M-8400/3 adenocarcinoma (T-173._)
M-8400/0 adenoma (T-173._)
M-8400/3 carcinoma (T-173._)
M-8400/1 tumor, NOS (T-173._)
M-8400/0 tumor, benign (T-173._)
M-8400/3 tumor, malignant (T-173._)

T-171.9 Sympathetic nervous system

M-8681/1 Sympathetic paraganglioma
M-9500/3 Sympathicoblastoma
M-9500/3 Sympathicogonioma
M-9500/3 Sympathogonioma

T-170.6 Symphysis pubis

M-9531/0 Syncytial meningioma (T-192._)
M-9701/3 Syndrome, Sezary's

T-171.9 Synovia, NOS

M------- Synovial chondromatosis (SNOMED M-73670)
M------- Synovial osteochondromatosis
(SNOMED M-73670)

Synovial sarcoma
M-9040/3 NOS
M-9043/3 biphasic type
M-9042/3 epithelioid cell type
M-9041/3 spindle cell type

Synovioma
M-9040/3 NOS
M-9040/0 benign
M-9040/3 malignant

M------- Synovitis, pigmented villonodular
(SNOMED M-47830)
M-8400/0 Syringadenoma, NOS (T-173._)
M-8406/0 Syringadenoma, papillary (T-173._)
M-8406/0 Syringocystadenoma, papillary (T-173._)
M-8407/0 Syringoma, NOS (T-173._)
M-8940/0 Syringoma, chondroid

Systemic
M------- hemangiomatosis (SNOMED M-76314)
M------- lymphangiomatosis (SNOMED M-76414)
M-9741/3 tissue mast cell disease

- T -

Tail
T-157.2 pancreas
T-174.6 breast
T-174.6 breast, axillary

T-191.8 Tapetum
T-170.8 Tarsal bone

M-9183/3 Telangiectatic osteosarcoma (T-170._)

Temple
T-173.3 NOS
T-173.3 NOS (carcinoma, melanoma, nevus)
T-171.0 NOS (sarcoma, lipoma)
T-171.0 adipose tissue
T-171.0 connective tissue
T-171.0 fatty tissue
T-171.0 fibrous tissue

Temple (Cont'd)

T-173.3	skin
T-171.0	soft tissue
T-171.0	subcutaneous tissue

T-170.0	Temporal bone
T-191.2	Temporal lobe
T-170.1	Temporomandibular joint

Tendon

T-171.9	NOS
T-171.3	ankle
T-171.2	arm
T-171.7	back
T-171.3	calf
T-171.2	finger
T-171.7	flank
T-171.3	foot
T-171.2	forearm
T-171.2	hand
T-171.3	heel
T-171.3	hip
T-171.3	knee
T-171.3	leg
T-171.0	neck
T-171.3	popliteal space
T-171.3	thigh
T-171.2	thumb
T-171.3	toe
T-171.2	wrist

Tendon sheath

T-171.9	NOS
T-171.3	ankle
T-171.2	arm
T-171.7	back
T-171.3	calf
T-171.2	finger
T-171.3	foot
T-171.2	forearm
T-171.2	hand
T-171.3	heel
T-171.3	hip
T-171.3	knee
T-171.3	leg
T-171.0	neck
T-171.3	popliteal space
T-171.3	thigh
T-171.2	thumb
T-171.3	toe
T-171.2	wrist

M-------	Tenosynovitis, nodular *(SNOMED M-478*
T-192.1	Tentorium, NOS
T-192.1	Tentorium cerebelli

M-9080/3	Teratoblastoma, malignant
M-9081/3	Teratocarcinoma
M-9502/3	Teratoid medulloepithelioma

Teratoma

M-9080/1	NOS
M-9080/0	adult, NOS
M-9080/0	adult, cystic
M-9081/3	and embryonal carcinoma, mixed
M-9080/0	benign
M-9101/3	combined with choriocarcinoma
M-9080/0	cystic, NOS
M-9080/0	cystic, adult
M-9080/0	differentiated type
M-9080/3	embryonal
M-9080/3	immature
M-9080/3	malignant, NOS
M-9082/3	malignant, anaplastic type
M-9083/3	malignant, intermediate type
M-9102/3	malignant, trophoblastic (T-186._)
M-9082/3	malignant, undifferentiated type
M-9080/0	mature
M-9080/1	solid

M-8250/3	Terminal bronchiolar carcinoma (T-162._)

T-186.9	Testicle, NOS

M-8640/0	Testicular adenoma
M-8590/1	Testicular stromal tumor (T-186._)

Testis

T-186.9	NOS
T-186.9	descended
T-186.0	ectopic *(site of neoplasm)*
T-186.0	retained *(site of neoplasm)*
T-186.9	scrotal
T-186.0	undescended *(site of neoplasm)*

T-191.0	Thalamus

Theca cell

M-8600/3	carcinoma (T-183.0)
M-8621/1	granulosa cell tumor (T-183.0)
M-8600/0	tumor (T-183.0)

M-8600/0 Thecoma, NOS **(T-183.0)**
M-8600/3 Thecoma, malignant **(T-183.0)**

Thigh
T-195.5   NOS
T-173.7   NOS (carcinoma, melanoma, nevus)
T-171.3   NOS (sarcoma, lipoma)
T-171.3   adipose tissue
T-171.3   connective tissue
T-171.3   fatty tissue
T-171.3   fibrous tissue
T-171.3   muscle
T-171.3   skeletal muscle
T-173.7   skin
T-171.3   soft tissue
T-171.3   subcutaneous tissue
T-171.3   tendon
T-171.3   tendon sheath

T-191.5   Third ventricle

Thoracic
T-192.2   cord
T-171.4   duct
T-150.1   esophagus
T-196.1   lymph node

Thoracic wall
T-195.1   NOS
T-173.5   NOS (carcinoma, melanoma, nevus)
T-171.4   NOS (sarcoma, lipoma)
T-171.4   adipose tissue
T-171.4   connective tissue
T-171.4   fatty tissue
T-171.4   fibrous tissue
T-171.4   muscle
T-171.4   skeletal muscle
T-173.5   skin
T-171.4   soft tissue
T-171.4   subcutaneous tissue

Thorax
T-195.1   NOS
T-171.4   connective tissue *(excludes Thymus, Heart and Mediastinum T-164._)*
T-171.4   muscle
T-171.4   skeletal muscle
T-173.5   skin
T-171.4   subcutaneous tissue

T-149.0   Throat

M-9962/1 Thrombocythemia, idiopathic **(T-169._)**
M-9910/3 Thrombocytic leukemia **(T-169._)**

Thumb
T-195.4   NOS
T-173.6   NOS (carcinoma, melanoma, nevus)
T-171.2   NOS (sarcoma, lipoma)
T-170.5   bone
T-171.2   connective tissue
T-171.2   fibrous tissue
T-171.2   muscle
T-171.2   skeletal muscle
T-173.6   skin
T-171.2   soft tissue
T-171.2   subcutaneous tissue
T-171.2   tendon
T-171.2   tendon sheath

M-8580/3 Thymic carcinoma **(T-164.0)**

Thymoma
M-8580/0   NOS **(T-164.0)**
M-8580/0   benign **(T-164.0)**
M-8580/3   malignant **(T-164.0)**

T-164.0   Thymus
T-193.9   Thyroglossal duct

M-------   Thyroglossal duct cyst *(SNOMED M-26500)*

Thyroid
T-193.9   NOS
T-161.3   cartilage
T-193.9   gland

T-170.7   Tibia

M-9261/3 Tibial adamantinoma **(T-170.7)**

T-196.5   Tibial lymph node
T-141.2   Tip of tongue

Toe
T-195.5   NOS
T-173.7   NOS (carcinoma, melanoma, nevus)
T-171.3   NOS (sarcoma, lipoma)
T-170.8   bone
T-171.3   connective tissue

Toe (Cont'd)

T-171.3	fibrous tissue
T-171.3	muscle
T-171.3	skeletal muscle
T-173.7	nail
T-173.7	skin
T-171.3	soft tissue
T-171.3	subcutaneous tissue
T-171.3	tendon
T-171.3	tendon sheath

Tongue

T-141.9	NOS
T-141.4	anterior, NOS
T-141.1	anterior, dorsal surface
T-141.3	anterior, ventral surface
T-141.4	anterior 2/3, NOS
T-141.1	anterior 2/3, dorsal surface
T-141.3	anterior 2/3, ventral surface
T-141.0	base, NOS
T-141.0	base, dorsal surface
T-141.2	border
T-141.1	dorsal surface, NOS
T-141.0	dorsal surface of base
T-141.3	frenulum linguae
T-141.5	junctional zone
T-141.9	lingual, NOS
T-141.6	lingual tonsil
T-141.1	midline
T-141.0	posterior, NOS
T-141.0	posterior third
T-141.0	root
T-141.2	tip
T-141.3	ventral surface, NOS
T-141.3	ventral surface, anterior
T-141.3	ventral surface, anterior 2/3

Tonsil

T-146.0	NOS *(excludes Lingual tonsil T-141.6 and Pharyngeal tonsil T-147.1)*
T-146.0	faucial
T-141.6	lingual
T-146.0	palatine
T-147.1	pharyngeal

T-146.1	Tonsillar fossa
T-146.2	Tonsillar pillar
T-143.9	Tooth socket

Trabecular

M-8190/3	adenocarcinoma

Trabecular (Cont'd)

M-8190/0	adenoma
M-8190/3	carcinoma
M-8332/3	type, follicular adenocarcinoma (T-193.9)
M-8332/3	type, follicular carcinoma (T-193.9)

T-162.0	Trachea
T-196.1	Tracheal lymph node
T-196.1	Tracheobronchial lymph node

Tract

T-159.9	alimentary, NOS
T-156.9	biliary, NOS
T-184.9	female genital, NOS
T-159.9	gastrointestinal, NOS
T-184.9	genitourinary, female, NOS
T-187.9	genitourinary, male, NOS
T-159.0	intestinal, NOS
T-187.9	male genital, NOS
T-192.0	optic
T-165.9	respiratory, NOS
T-165.0	upper respiratory
T-190.0	uveal

T-173.2	Tragus

Transitional

M-8120/3	carcinoma
M-9537/0	meningioma (T-192._)
M-8120/0	papilloma

Transitional cell carcinoma

M-8120/3	NOS
M-8120/2	in-situ
M-8130/3	papillary
M-8122/3	spindle cell type

M-8120/0	Transitional cell papilloma, NOS
M-8121/1	Transitional cell papilloma, inverted type

T-153.1	Transverse colon
T-171.4	Trapezius muscle

M-------	Traumatic neuroma *(SNOMED M-49770)*

T-145.6	Triangle, retromolar
T-171.2	Triceps brachii muscle

M-8100/0	Trichoepithelioma (T-173._)
M-8101/0	Trichofolliculoma (T-173._)
M-8102/0	Tricholemmoma (T-173._)

		Tumor (Cont'd)	
T-192.0	Trigeminal nerve	M-8390/0	adnexal (T-173._)
T-145.6	Trigone, retromolar	M-8370/0	adrenal cortical, NOS (T-194.0)
T-188.0	Trigone, urinary bladder	M-8370/0	adrenal cortical, benign (T-194.0)
T-192.0	Trochlear nerve	M-8370/3	adrenal cortical, malignant (T-194.0)
		M-8671/0	adrenal rest
M-9102/3	Trophoblastic malignant teratoma (T-186._)	M-8152/3	alpha-cell, malignant (T-157._)
		M-------	amyloid (SNOMED M-55160)
T-161.0	True cord	M-8691/1	aortic body (T-194.6)
T-161.0	True vocal cord	M-8090/1	basal cell (T-173._)
		M-8000/0	benign
		M-8000/0	benign, unclassified
	Trunk	M-8151/3	beta-cell, malignant (T-157._)
T-195.8	NOS	M-9000/0	Brenner, NOS (T-183.0)
T-173.5	NOS (carcinoma, melanoma, nevus)	M-9000/1	Brenner, borderline malignancy (T-183.0)
T-171.7	NOS (sarcoma, lipoma)	M-9000/3	Brenner, malignant (T-183.0)
T-171.7	adipose tissue	M-9000/1	Brenner, proliferating (T-183.0)
T-171.7	connective tissue	M-8100/0	Brooke's (T-173._)
T-171.7	fatty tissue	M-8880/0	brown fat
T-171.7	fibrous tissue	M-9750/3	Burkitt's
T-171.7	muscle	M-8240/1	carcinoid, NOS
T-171.7	skeletal muscle	M-8241/1	carcinoid, argentaffin, NOS
T-173.5	skin	M-8241/3	carcinoid, argentaffin, malignant
T-171.7	soft tissue	M-8240/3	carcinoid, malignant
T-171.7	subcutaneous tissue	M-8242/1	carcinoid, non-argentaffin, NOS
		M-8242/3	carcinoid, non-argentaffin, malignant
		M-8692/1	carotid body (T-194.5)
	Tube	M-8001/1	cells, NOS
T-160.1	auditory	M-8001/0	cells, benign
T-160.1	Eustachian	M-8001/3	cells, malignant
T-183.2	fallopian	M-8001/1	cells, uncertain whether benign or malignant
T-183.2	uterine		
		M-8700/0	chromaffin
T-183.8	Tubo-ovarian	M-9230/0	Codman's (T-170._)
		M-8000/6	embolus
		M-9071/3	endodermal sinus
	Tubular	M-8010/0	epithelial, benign
M-8211/3	adenocarcinoma	M-8010/3	epithelial, malignant
M-8211/0	adenoma, NOS	M-9260/3	Ewing's (T-170._)
M-8210/3	adenoma, adenocarcinoma in	M-8004/3	fusiform cell type, malignant
M-8640/0	adenoma, Pick's	M-8153/1	G cell, NOS
M-8640/0	androblastoma, NOS	M-8153/3	G cell, malignant
M-8641/0	androblastoma with lipid storage (T-183.0)	M-9250/1	giant cell, bone, NOS (T-170._)
M-8211/3	carcinoma	M-9250/3	giant cell, bone, malignant (T-170._)
		M-9230/0	giant cell, chondromatous (T-170._)
M-8263/0	Tubulovillous adenoma	M-9251/1	giant cell, soft parts, NOS
		M-9251/3	giant cell, soft parts, malignant
		M-------	giant cell, tendon sheath (SNOMED M-47830)
	Tumor	M-8003/3	giant cell type, malignant
M-8000/1	NOS	M-8711/0	glomus
M-8550/1	acinar cell	M-8690/1	glomus jugulare (T-194.6)
M-8550/1	acinic cell	M-8590/1	gonadal stromal
M-9054/0	adenomatoid, NOS	M-9580/0	granular cell, NOS
M-9300/0	adenomatoid, odontogenic		

Tumor (Cont'd)

M-9580/3	granular cell, malignant
M-8620/1	granulosa cell, NOS (T-183.0)
M-8620/3	granulosa cell, malignant (T-183.0)
M-8621/1	granulosa cell-theca cell (T-183.0)
M-8312/3	Grawitz (T-189.0)
M-8660/0	hilar cell (T-183.0)
M-8290/0	Hürthle cell (T-193.9)
M-8311/1	hypernephroid
M-8650/1	interstitial cell, NOS
M-8650/0	interstitial cell, benign
M-8650/3	interstitial cell, malignant
M-8150/0	islet cell (T-157._)
M-8361/1	juxtaglomerular (T-189.0)
M-8490/6	Krukenberg (T-183.0)
M-8650/1	Leydig cell, NOS (T-186._)
M-8650/0	Leydig cell, benign (T-186._)
M-8650/3	Leydig cell, malignant (T-186._)
M-8670/0	lipid cell, ovary (T-183.0)
M-8670/0	lipoid cell, ovary (T-183.0)
M-9590/0	lymphomatous, benign
M-8000/3	malignant, NOS
M-8004/3	malignant, fusiform cell type
M-8003/3	malignant, giant cell type
M-8940/3	malignant, mixed, NOS
M-8940/3	malignant, mixed, salivary gland type
M-8002/3	malignant, small cell type
M-8004/3	malignant, spindle cell type
M-8000/3	malignant, unclassified
M-9740/1	mast cell, NOS
M-9740/3	mast cell, malignant
M-9363/0	melanotic neuroectodermal
M-8800/3	mesenchymal, malignant
M-8951/3	mesodermal, mixed
M-9110/1	mesonephric
M-8000/6	metastatic
M-8940/0	mixed, NOS
M-8940/3	mixed, malignant, NOS
M-8990/1	mixed, mesenchymal
M-8951/3	mixed, mesodermal
M-8940/0	mixed, salivary gland type, NOS
M-8940/3	mixed, salivary gland type, malignant
M-8243/3	mucocarcinoid, malignant
M-8430/1	mucoepidermoid
M-8950/3	Müllerian mixed
M-8982/0	myoepithelial
M-8350/3	nonencapsulated sclerosing (T-193.9)
M-9270/1	odontogenic, NOS (T-170._)
M-9300/0	odontogenic, adenomatoid (T-170._)
M-9270/0	odontogenic, benign (T-170._)
M-9340/0	odontogenic, calcifying epithelial (T-170._)
M-9270/3	odontogenic, malignant (T-170._)
M-9312/0	odontogenic, squamous (T-170._)

Tumor (Cont'd)

M-9520/3	olfactory, neurogenic
M-8590/1	ovarian stromal (T-183.0)
M-9507/0	Pacinian
M-9731/1	plasma cell, NOS
M-9731/0	plasma cell, benign
M-9731/3	plasma cell, malignant
M-9071/3	polyvesicular vitelline
M-9350/1	Rathke's pouch (T-194.3)
M-9363/0	retinal anlage
M-8000/6	secondary
M-8640/0	Sertoli cell, NOS
M-8641/0	Sertoli cell with lipid storage
M-8631/0	Sertoli-Leydig cell
M-8590/1	sex cord
M-8590/1	sex cord-stromal
M-8390/0	skin appendage (T-173._)
M-8002/3	small cell type, malignant
M-8800/0	soft tissue, benign
M-8800/3	soft tissue, malignant
M-8004/3	spindle cell type, malignant
M-8400/1	sweat gland, NOS (T-173._)
M-8400/0	sweat gland, benign (T-173._)
M-8400/3	sweat gland, malignant (T-173._)
M-8590/1	testicular stromal (T-186._)
M-8600/0	theca cell (T-183.0)
M-8621/1	theca cell-granulosa cell (T-183.0)
M-8200/0	turban (T-173.4)
M-8561/0	Warthin's (T-142._)
M-8960/3	Wilms's (T-189.0)
M-9071/3	yolk sac

Tumor, unclassified

M-8000/0	benign
M-8000/3	malignant
M-8000/9	malignant, uncertain whether primary or metastatic
M-8000/1	uncertain whether benign or malignant

M-------	Tumoral calcinosis (*SNOMED M-55520*)
M-8041/1	Tumorlet
T-187.8	Tunica vaginalis
M-8200/0	Turban tumor (T-173.4)
T-160.0	Turbinate, nasal
T-160.1	Tympanic cavity

- U -

M-8090/3 Ulcer, rodent (T-173._)

T-170.4 Ulna
T-171.2 Ulnar artery
T-171.2 Ulnar nerve

Umbilicus
T-173.5 NOS
T-173.5 NOS (carcinoma, melanoma, nevus)
T-171.5 NOS (sarcoma, lipoma)
T-171.5 connective tissue
T-171.5 fibrous tissue
T-173.5 skin
T-171.5 soft tissue
T-171.5 subcutaneous tissue

M-____/1 Uncertain whether benign or malignant (see Behavior code, page 20)
M-____/9 Uncertain whether primary or metastatic (see Behavior code, page 20)

Unclassified tumor
M-8000/0 benign
M-8000/3 malignant
M-8000/9 malignant, uncertain whether primary or metastatic
M-8000/1 uncertain whether benign or malignant

T-191.2 Uncus
T-186.0 Undescended testis (site of neoplasm)

M-____/.(4) Undifferentiated (see Grading code, page 20)

Undifferentiated type
M-8020/3 carcinoma, NOS
M-9082/3 malignant teratoma
M-9512/3 retinoblastoma (T-190.5)

T-199.9 Unknown primary site

Upper
T-143.0 alveolar mucosa
T-143.0 alveolar ridge mucosa
T-143.0 alveolus
T-174.8 breast
T-143.0 gingiva
T-143.0 gum

Upper (Cont'd)
T-174.2 inner quadrant of breast
T-170.0 jaw bone
T-173.1 lid
T-140.0 lip, NOS (excludes Skin of upper lip T-173.0)
T-140.0 lip, external
T-140.3 lip, frenulum
T-140.3 lip, inner aspect
T-140.3 lip, mucosa
T-173.0 lip, skin
T-140.0 lip, vermilion border
T-162.3 lobe, bronchus
T-162.3 lobe, lung
T-174.4 outer quadrant of breast
T-165.0 respiratory tract
T-150.3 third of esophagus

Upper limb
T-195.4 NOS
T-173.6 NOS (carcinoma, melanoma, nevus)
T-171.2 NOS (sarcoma, lipoma)
T-171.2 adipose tissue
T-171.2 connective tissue
T-171.2 fatty tissue
T-171.2 fibrous tissue
T-170.4 long bone
T-170.4 long bones, joints
T-196.3 lymph node
T-171.2 muscle
T-171.2 skeletal muscle
T-170.5 short bone
T-170.5 short bones, joints
T-173.6 skin
T-171.2 soft tissue
T-171.2 subcutaneous tissue
T-171.2 tendon
T-171.2 tendon sheath

T-188.7 Urachus
T-189.2 Ureter
T-188.6 Ureteric orifice
T-189.3 Urethra
T-189.3 Urethral gland
T-188.5 Urethral orifice, internal
T-184.9 Urethrovaginal septum

Urinary bladder
T-188.9 NOS
T-188.3 anterior wall
T-188.1 dome
T-188.5 internal urethral orifice

Urinary bladder (Cont'd)

T-188.2	lateral wall
T-188.5	neck
T-188.4	posterior wall
T-188.0	trigone
T-188.7	urachus
T-188.6	ureteric orifice
T-188.9	wall, NOS
T-188.3	wall, anterior
T-188.2	wall, lateral
T-188.4	wall, posterior

T-189.9	Urinary system, NOS

M-8120/3	Urothelial carcinoma
M-8120/1	Urothelial papilloma

Uterine

T-179.9	NOS
T-183.9	adnexa
T-180.9	cervix
T-183.4	ligament
T-182.1	lower segment
T-183.2	tube

T-183.8	Utero-ovarian
T-183.4	Uterosacral ligament

Uterus

T-179.9	NOS
T-183.9	adnexa, NOS
T-183.9	adnexa, uterine
T-182.0	body
T-180.0	cervical canal
T-180.8	cervical stump
T-180.9	cervix, NOS
T-180.8	cervix, squamocolumnar junction
T-180.9	cervix uteri
T-182.0	corpus uteri
T-180.0	endocervical canal
T-180.0	endocervical gland
T-180.0	endocervix
T-182.0	endometrial gland
T-182.0	endometrial stroma
T-182.0	endometrium
T-180.1	exocervix
T-180.1	external os
T-181.9	fetal membranes
T-182.0	fundus uteri
T-180.0	internal os
T-182.1	isthmus uteri

Uterus (Cont'd)

T-183.3	ligament, broad
T-183.5	ligament, round
T-183.4	ligament, uterine
T-183.4	ligament, uterosacral
T-182.1	lower uterine segment
T-182.0	myometrium
T-180.0	Nabothian gland
T-183.4	parametrium
T-181.9	placenta
T-180.8	squamocolumnar junction of cervix
T-183.9	uterine adnexa
T-180.9	uterine cervix

T-189.3	Utricle, prostatic
T-190.0	Uveal tract
T-145.4	Uvula

- V -

T-184.0	Vagina, NOS
T-184.0	Vagina, fornix
T-184.0	Vaginal vault
T-192.0	Vagus nerve
T-146.3	Vallecula, NOS
T-146.3	Vallecula epiglottica
T-153.4	Valve, ileocecal
T-187.6	Vas deferens

Vascular

M-8894/0	leiomyoma
M-------	nevus (SNOMED M-75540)
M-------	spider (SNOMED M-76330)

T-184.0	Vault, vaginal
T-171.9	Vein, NOS
T-171.6	Vein, iliac

Vena cava

T-171.5	NOS
T-171.5	abdominal
T-171.5	inferior
T-171.4	superior

M-9122/0	Venous hemangioma

Ventral surface of tongue

T-141.3	NOS
T-141.3	anterior
T-141.3	anterior 2/3

Ventricle

T-191.5	NOS
T-164.1	cardiac
T-191.5	cerebral
T-191.5	fourth
T-191.5	lateral
T-191.5	third

T-161.1 Ventricular band of larynx

Vermilion border

T-140.9	lip, NOS
T-140.1	lower lip
T-140.0	upper lip

T-191.6 Vermis of cerebellum

Verruca

M-------	NOS (SNOMED M-76600)
M-------	plana (SNOMED M-76620)
M-------	seborrheic (SNOMED M-72750)
M-------	vulgaris (SNOMED M-76630)

Verrucous

M-8051/3	carcinoma, NOS
M-8051/3	carcinoma, epidermoid
M-8051/3	carcinoma, squamous cell
M-9142/0	keratotic hemangioma
M-8051/0	papilloma

T-170.2	Vertebra
T-170.2	Vertebral column (excludes Sacrum and Coccyx T-170.6)
T-187.8	Vesicle, seminal
T-184.9	Vesicocervical tissue
T-184.9	Vesicovaginal septum
T-171.9	Vessel, NOS
T-145.1	Vestibule of mouth
T-160.0	Vestibule of nose

M-8263/0	Villoglandular adenoma
M-------	Villonodular pigmented synovitis (SNOMED M-47830)

Villous

M-8262/3	adenocarcinoma
M-8261/1	adenoma, NOS
M-8261/3	adenoma, adenocarcinoma in
M-8261/1	papilloma

T-163.1 Visceral pleura

Vocal cord

T-161.0	NOS
T-161.1	false
T-161.0	true

M-------	von Recklinghausen's disease, bone (SNOMED M-74840)
M-9540/1	von Recklinghausen's disease (except of Bone)

T-184.4	Vulva, NOS
T-184.4	Vulva, skin

- W -

T-149.1 Waldeyer's ring, NOS

M-------	Walthard's rest (SNOMED M-26350)
M-8561/0	Warthin's tumor (T-142.__)

Water-clear cell

M-8322/3	adenocarcinoma (T-194.1)
M-8322/0	adenoma (T-194.1)
M-8322/3	carcinoma (T-194.1)

M-___/_.(1) Well differentiated (see Grading code, page 20)

Well differentiated type

M-8331/3	follicular adenocarcinoma (T-193.9)
M-8331/3	follicular carcinoma (T-193.9)
M-8851/3	liposarcoma

T-142.1	Wharton's duct
T-191.0	White matter, central
T-191.0	White matter, cerebral

M-8960/3 Wilms's tumor (T-189.0)

T-157.3 Wirsung's duct

M-9110/0 Wolffian duct adenoma
M-9110/3 Wolffian duct carcinoma

Wrist
T-195.4 NOS
T-173.6 NOS (carcinoma, melanoma, nevus)
T-171.2 NOS (sarcoma, lipoma)
T-170.5 bone
T-171.2 connective tissue
T-171.2 fibrous tissue
T-170.5 joint
T-173.6 skin
T-171.2 soft tissue
T-171.2 subcutaneous tissue
T-171.2 tendon
T-171.2 tendon sheath

M-8332/3 Wuchernde Struma Langhans **(T-193.9)**

- X -

M-8831/0 Xanthofibroma
M------- Xanthogranuloma, NOS *(SNOMED M-44040)*
M------- Xanthogranuloma, juvenile
          (SNOMED M-55380)
M------- Xanthoma, NOS *(SNOMED M-55300)*
M------- Xeroderma pigmentosum *(SNOMED M-74040)*

- Y -

M-9071/3 Yolk sac tumor

- Z -

T-154.8 Zone, cloacogenic
T-141.5 Zone, junctional of tongue
T-194.6 Zuckerkandl's organ
T-170.0 Zygomatic bone

- 128 -

TUMOR-LIKE LESIONS AND CONDITIONS

Acanthosis nigricans
Actinic keratosis
Adenofibrosis
Adenoma sebaceum
Adenomatous goiter
Adenomatous hyperplasia
Adenomyomatous hyperplasia
Adenomyosis, NOS
Adenosis, NOS
Amputation neuroma
Amyloid tumor
Aneurysmal bone cyst
Angio-immunoblastic lymphadenopathy
Angiomatosis, NOS
Angiomatous lymphoid hamartoma
Atrophy-associated hyperplasia
Atypical hyperplasia

Basal cell papilloma
Basosquamous papilloma
Benign angiofollicular hyperplasia
Benign lymphocytic infiltrate of Jessner
Benign lymphocytoma cutis
Benign lymphoepithelial lesion
Benign lymphoid polyp
Benign squamous keratosis
Birthmark

Central giant cell granuloma
Chalazion
Cholesteatoma, NOS
Choristoma
Cicatricial fibromatosis
Clear cell acanthoma
Colitis cystica profunda
Colloid goiter
Condyloma, NOS
Condyloma acuminatum
Congenital cyst, NOS
Congenital dysplasia, NOS
Congenital melanosis
Cutaneous horn
Cyst, NOS
Cystic disease of breast
Cystitis cystica

Decidual change
Dentigerous cyst

Diffuse lipomatosis
Dysgenesis, NOS
Dysplasia, NOS
Dysplasia, mild
Dysplasia, moderate
Dysplasia, severe

Ectopia, NOS
Ectopic glial tissue
Embryonal rest, NOS
Endemic goiter
Endometrioma
Endometriosis, NOS
Enterogenous cyst
Eosinophilic granuloma, NOS
Eosinophilic granuloma of bone
Ephelis
Epidermoid cholesteatoma
Epidermoid cyst
Eruption cyst
Exostosis, NOS
External endometriosis

Fat necrosis
Fibrocystic disease, NOS
Fibroepithelial papilloma
Fibroepithelial polyp
Fibromatosis, NOS
Fibrosclerosis
Fibrosing adenomatosis
Fibrosing adenosis
Fibrosis, NOS
Fibrous dysplasia, NOS
Fibrous polyp
Florid adenosis
Focal nodular hyperplasia
Follicular cyst of jaw
Fordyce's disease
Freckle, NOS

Ganglion cyst
Giant cell reparative granuloma
Giant cell tumor of tendon sheath
Giant condyloma
Giant rugal hypertrophy
Gingival cyst, NOS
Gingival odontogenic cyst
Glandular and stromal hyperplasia

Glandular hyperplasia
Glandular metaplasia
Goiter, NOS
Granuloma, NOS
Granuloma pyogenicum
Gynecomastia

Hamartoma, NOS
Hand-Schüller-Christian disease
Hemangioma of granulation tissue type
Hemangiomatosis, NOS
Hematoma, NOS
Heterotopia, NOS
Histiocytosis, NOS
Histiocytosis X, NOS
Hyperplasia, NOS
Hyperplastic polyp
Hyperplastic scar
Hyperthecosis
Hypertrophy, NOS

Immunoblastic lymphadenopathy
Infiltrative fasciitis
Inflammatory polyp
Inflammatory pseudotumor
Internal endometriosis
Inverted follicular keratosis

Juvenile aponeurotic fibroma
Juvenile polyp
Juvenile xanthogranuloma

Keloid
Keratoacanthoma, NOS
Keratocyst
Keratosis, NOS
Keratosis obturans

Lentigo, NOS
Leucokeratosis
Leucoplakia, NOS
Lipogranuloma, NOS
Lipomatosis, NOS
Lobular hyperplasia
Lymphoid hyperplasia, NOS
Lymphoid polyp, NOS
Lymphomatoid papulosis

Malakoplakia
Mammary duct ectasia
Mesenchymal hamartoma
Metaphyseal fibrous defect
Metaplasia, NOS
Metaplastic polyp

Molluscum contagiosum
Molluscum sebaceum
Mucocele
Musculo-aponeurotic fibromatosis
Myelofibrosis
Myeloid metaplasia
Myelosclerosis, NOS
Myositis ossificans, NOS

Nasal glial heterotopia
Nasal glioma
Nasopalatine duct cyst
Nevoxanthoendothelioma
Nevus araneus
Nevus flammeus
Nevus sanguineus
Nevus sebaceus of Jadassohn
Nevus unius lateris
Nevus verrucosus
Nodular fasciitis
Nodular hyperplasia, NOS
Nodular tenosynovitis
Non-ossifying fibroma

Odontogenic cyst, NOS
Odontogenic cyst, dentigerous
Odontogenic cyst, eruptive
Odontogenic cyst, gingival
Odontogenic cyst, primordial
Oncocytosis
Orbital lymphoma
Osteitis deformans
Osteitis fibrosa cystica

Paget's disease of bone
Papillary cystitis
Papilliferous hyperplasia
Periapical cemental dysplasia
Peripheral odontogenic fibroma
Peutz-Jeghers polyp
Pigmented villonodular synovitis
Pilar cyst
Plasma cell granuloma
Plasma cell pseudotumor
Polycythemia, secondary
Polyp, NOS
Portwine nevus
Pregnancy luteoma
Primordial cyst
Pseudoepitheliomatous hyperplasia
Pseudolymphoma
Pseudopolyp, NOS
Pseudosarcoma
Pseudosarcomatous fasciitis

Pseudosarcomatous fibromatosis
Pseudotumor, NOS
Pyogenic granuloma

Radicular cyst
Reticulohistiocytic granuloma
Reticulohistiocytoma

Salpingitis isthmica nodosa
Sarcoid granuloma
Sclerosing adenosis
Sebaceous cyst
Seborrheic keratosis
Seborrheic verruca
Senile keratosis
Sinus histiocytosis with massive
    lymphadenopathy
Solitary cyst
Spider angioma
Spider nevus
Spongy nevus of mucosa
Squamous metaplasia
Steatocystoma multiplex

Strawberry nevus
Stromal hyperplasia
Synovial chondromatosis
Synovial osteochondromatosis
Systemic hemangiomatosis
Systemic lymphangiomatosis

Thyroglossal duct cyst
Traumatic neuroma
Tumoral calcinosis

Vascular nevus
Vascular spider
Verruca, NOS
Verruca plana
Verruca vulgaris
von Recklinghausen's disease of bone

Walthard's rest

Xanthogranuloma, NOS
Xanthoma, NOS
Xeroderma pigmentosum

WHO publications may be obtained, direct or through booksellers, from:

ALGERIA : Société nationale d'Edition et de Diffusion, 3 bd Zirout Youcef, ALGIERS

ARGENTINA : Librería de las Naciones, Cooperativa Ltda, Alsina 500, BUENOS AIRES — Editorial Sudamericana S.A., Humberto 1º 545, BUENOS AIRES

AUSTRALIA : Mail Order Sales, Australian Government Publishing Service, P.O. Box 84, CANBERRA A.C.T. 2600 ; *or over the counter from* Australian Government Publications and Inquiry Centres at : 113 London Circuit, CANBERRA CITY ; 347 Swanston Street, MELBOURNE ; 309 Pitt Street, SYDNEY ; Mr. Newman House, 200 St. George's Terrace, PERTH ; Industry House, 12 Pirie Street, ADELAIDE ; 156-162 Macquarie Street, HOBART — Hunter Publications, 58a Gipps Street, COLLINGWOOD, Vic. 3066

AUSTRIA : Gerold & Co., I. Graben 31, VIENNA 1

BANGLADESH : WHO Representative, G.P.O. Box 250, DACCA 5

BELGIUM : Office international de Librairie, 30 avenue Marnix, BRUSSELS

BRAZIL : Biblioteca Regional de Medicina OMS/OPS, Unidad de Venta de Publicaciones, Caixa Postal 20.381, Vila Clementino, 01000 São Paulo — S.P.

BURMA : *see* India, WHO Regional Office

CANADA : Information Canada Bookstore, 171 Slater Street, OTTAWA, Ontario K1A 0S9 ; Main Library, University of Calgary, CALGARY, Alberta ; 1683 Barrington Street, HALIFAX, N.S. B3J 1Z9 ; 640 Ste Catherine West, MONTREAL, Quebec H3B 1B8 ; 221 Yonge Street, TORONTO, Ontario M5B 1N4 ; 800 Granville Street, VANCOUVER, B.C. V6Z 1K4 ; 393 Portage Avenue, WINNIPEG, Manitoba R3B 2C6. *Mail orders to* 171 Slater Street, OTTAWA, Ontario K1A 0S9

CHINA : China National Publications Import Corporation, P.O. Box 88, PEKING

COLOMBIA : Distrilibros Ltda, Pío Alfonso García, Carrera 4a, Nos 36-119, CARTAGENA

COSTA RICA : Imprenta y Librería Trejos S.A., Apartado 1313, SAN JOSÉ

CYPRUS : MAM, P.O. Box 1674, NICOSIA

CZECHOSLOVAKIA : Artia, Smecky 30, 111 27 PRAGUE 1

DENMARK : Ejnar Munksgaard, Ltd, Nørregade 6, COPENHAGEN

ECUADOR : Librería Científica S.A., P.O. Box 362, Luque 223, GUAYAQUIL

EGYPT : Nabaa El Fikr Bookshop, 55 Saad Zaghloul Street, ALEXANDRIA — Anglo Egyptian Bookshop, 165 Mohamed Farid Street, CAIRO

EL SALVADOR : Librería Estudiantil Edificio Comercial B No 3, Avenida Libertad, SAN SALVADOR

FIJI : The WHO Representative, P.O. Box 113, SUVA

FINLAND : Akateeminen Kirjakauppa, Keskuskatu 2, HELSINKI 10

FRANCE : Librairie Arnette, 2 rue Casimir-Delavigne, PARIS 6e

GERMAN DEMOCRATIC REPUBLIC : Buchhaus Leipzig, Postfach 140, 701 LEIPZIG

GERMANY, FEDERAL REPUBLIC OF : Govi-Verlag GmbH, Ginnheimerstrasse 20, Postfach 5360, 6236 ESCHBORN — W. E. Saarbach, Postfach 1510, Follerstrasse 2, 5 COLOGNE 1 — Alex. Horn, Spiegelgasse 9, Postfach 3340, 62 WIESBADEN

GREECE : G. C. Eleftheroudakis S.A., Librairie internationale, rue Nikis 4, ATHENS (T. 126)

HAITI : Max Bouchereau, Librairie "A la Caravelle ", Boîte postale 111-B, PORT-AU-PRINCE

HUNGARY : Kultura, P.O.B. 149, BUDAPEST 62 — Akadémiai Könyvesbolt, Váci utca 22, BUDAPEST V

ICELAND : Snaebjørn Jonsson & Co., P.O. Box 1131, Hafnarstraeti 9, REYKJAVIK

INDIA : WHO Regional Office for South-East Asia, World Health House, Indraprastha Estate, Ring Road, NEW DELHI 1 — Oxford Book & Stationery Co., Scindia House, NEW DELHI ; 17 Park Street, CALCUTTA 16 (Sub-Agent)

INDONESIA : *see* India, WHO Regional Office

IRAN : Iranian Amalgamated Distribution Agency, 151 Khiaban Soraya, TEHERAN

IRELAND : The Stationery Office, DUBLIN

ISRAEL : Heiliger & Co., 3 Nathan Strauss Street, JERUSALEM

ITALY : Edizioni Minerva Medica, Corso Bramante 83-85, TURIN ; Via Lamarmora 3, MILAN

JAPAN : Maruzen Company, Ltd, P.O. Box 5050, TOKYO International, 100-31

KENYA : The Caxton Press Ltd, Head Office : Gathani House, Huddersfield Road, P.O. Box 1742, NAIROBI

KUWAIT : The Kuwait Bookshops Co. Ltd, Thunayan Al-Ghanem Bldg, P.O. Box 2942, KUWAIT

LAO PEOPLE'S DEMOCRATIC REPUBLIC : The WHO Representative, P.O. Box 343, VIENTIANE

LEBANON : Documenta Scientifica/Redico, P.O. Box 5641, BEIRUT

LUXEMBOURG : Librairie du Centre, 49 bd Royal, LUXEMBOURG

MALAYSIA : The WHO Representative, Room 1004, Fitzpatrick Building, Jalan Raja Chulan, KUALA LUMPUR 05-02 — Jubilee (Book) Store Ltd. 97 Jalan Tuanku Abdul Rahman, P.O. Box 629, KUALA LUMPUR — Parry's Book Center, K.L. Hilton Hotel, KUALA LUMPUR

MEXICO : La Prensa Médica Mexicana, Ediciones Científicas, Paseo de las Facultades 26, MEXICO CITY 20, D.F.

MONGOLIA : *see* India, WHO Regional Office

MOROCCO : Editions La Porte, 281 avenue Mohammed V, RABAT

NEPAL : *see* India, WHO Regional Office

NETHERLANDS : N. V. Martinus Nijhoff's Boekhandel en Uitgevers Maatschappij, Lange Voorhout 9, THE HAGUE

NEW ZEALAND : Government Printing Office, Government Bookshops at : Rutland Street, P.O. Box 5344, AUCKLAND ; 130 Oxford Terrace, P.O. Box 1721, CHRISTCHURCH ; Alma Street, P.O. Box 857, HAMILTON ; Princes Street, P.O. Box 1104, DUNEDIN ; Mulgrave Street, Private Bag, WELLINGTON — R. Hill & Son, Ltd, Ideal House, Cnr. Gilles Avenue & Eden St., Newmarket, AUCKLAND S.E.1

NIGERIA : University Bookshop Nigeria, Ltd, University of Ibadan, IBADAN

NORWAY : Johan Grundt Tanum Bokhandel, Karl Johansgt. 43, OSLO 1

PAKISTAN : Mirza Book Agency, 65 Shahrah Quaid-E. Azam, P.O. Box 729, LAHORE 3

PARAGUAY : Agencia de Librerías Nizza S.A., Estrella No. 721, ASUNCIÓN

PERU : Distribuidora Inca S.A., Apartado 3115, Emilio Althaus 470, LIMA

PHILIPPINES : World Health Organization, Regional Office for the Western Pacific, P.O. Box 2932, MANILA — The Modern Book Company Inc., P.O. Box 632, 926 Rizal Avenue, MANILA

POLAND : Składnica Księgarska, ul. Mazowiecka 9, WARSAW (*except periodicals*) — BKWZ Ruch, ul. Wronia 23, WARSAW (*periodicals only*)

PORTUGAL : Livraria Rodrigues, 186 Rua Aurea, LISBON

REPUBLIC OF KOREA : The WHO Representative, Central P.O. Box 540, SEOUL

SINGAPORE : The WHO Representative, 144 Moulmein Road, G.P.O. Box 3457, SINGAPORE 1

SOUTH AFRICA : Van Schalk's Bookstore (Pty) Ltd, P.O. Box 724, PRETORIA

SPAIN : Comercial Atheneum S.A., Consejo de Ciento 130-136, BARCELONA 15 ; General Moscardó 29, MADRID 20 — Librería Díaz de Santos, Lagasca 95, MADRID 6

SRI LANKA : *see* India, WHO Regional Office

SWEDEN : Aktiebolaget C. E. Fritzes Kungl. Hovbokhandel, Fredsgatan 2, STOCKHOLM 16

SWITZERLAND : Medizinischer Verlag Hans Huber, Länggass Strasse 76, 3012 BERNE 9

THAILAND : *see* India, WHO Regional Office

TUNISIA : Société Tunisienne de Diffusion, 5 avenue de Carthage, TUNIS

TURKEY : Librairie Hachette, 469 av. de l'Indépendance, ISTANBUL

UGANDA : *see address under* KENYA

UNITED KINGDOM : H. M. Stationery Office : 49 High Holborn, LONDON WC1V 6HB ; 13a Castle Street, EDINBURGH EH2 3AR ; 41 The Hayes, CARDIFF CF1 1JW ; 80 Chichester Street, BELFAST BT1 4JY ; Brazennose Street, MANCHESTER M60 8AS ; 258 Broad Street, BIRMINGHAM B1 2HE ; Southey House, Wine Street, BRISTOL BS1 2BQ. *All mail orders should be sent to* P.O. Box 569, LONDON SE1 9NH

UNITED REPUBLIC OF TANZANIA : *see address under* KENYA

UNITED STATES OF AMERICA : *Single and bulk copies of individual publications (Not subscriptions) :* Q Corporation, 49 Sheridan Avenue, ALBANY, NY 12210. *Subscriptions :* Subscription orders, accompanied by check made out to the Chemical Bank, NEW YORK, Account World Health Organization, should be sent to the World Health Organization, P.O. Box 5284, Church Street Station, NEW YORK, NY 10249. Correspondence concerning subscriptions should be forwarded to the World Health Organization, Distribution and Sales Service, 1211 GENEVA 27, Switzerland. *Publications are also available from the* United Nations Bookshop, NEW YORK, NY 10017 (*retail only*)

USSR : *For readers in the USSR requiring Russian editions :* Komsomolskij prospekt 18, Medicinskaja Kniga, Moscow — *For readers outside the USSR requiring Russian editions :* Kuzneckij most 18, Meždunarodnaja Kniga, Moscow G-200

VENEZUELA : Editorial Interamericana de Venezuela C.A., Apartado 50785, CARACAS — Librería del Este, Av. Francisco de Miranda 52, Edificio Galipán, CARACAS

YUGOSLAVIA : Jugoslovenska Knjiga, Terazije 27/II, BELGRADE

Orders from countries where sales agents have not yet been appointed may be addressed to

World Health Organization, Distribution and Sales Service, 1211 Geneva 27, Switzerland,

but must be paid for in pounds sterling, US dollars or Swiss francs.